Pharmacologic Support in Pain Management

Editors

STEVEN STANOS
JAMES R. BABINGTON

PHYSICAL MEDICINE AND REHABILITATION CLINICS OF NORTH AMERICA

www.pmr.theclinics.com

Consulting Editor
SANTOS F. MARTINEZ

May 2020 • Volume 31 • Number 2

ELSEVIER

1600 John F. Kennedy Boulevard • Suite 1800 • Philadelphia, Pennsylvania, 19103-2899

http://www.theclinics.com

PHYSICAL MEDICINE AND REHABILITATION CLINICS OF NORTH AMERICA Volume 31, Number 2
May 2020 ISSN 1047-9651, ISBN 978-0-323-73370-0

Editor: Lauren Boyle
Developmental Editor: Nicole Congleton

Reprints. For copies of 100 or more of articles in this publication, please contact the Commercial Reprints Department, Elsevier Inc., 360 Park Avenue South, New York, NY 10010-1710. Tel.: 212-633-3874; Fax: 212-633-3820; E-mail: reprints@elsevier.com.

Physical Medicine and Rehabilitation Clinics of North America (ISSN 1047-9651) is published quarterly by Elsevier Inc., 360 Park Avenue South, New York, NY 10010-1710. Months of issue are February, May, August, and November. Business and Editorial Offices: 1600 John F. Kennedy Blvd., Suite 1800, Philadelphia, PA 19103-2899. Customer Service Office: 3251 Riverport Lane, Maryland Heights, MO 63043. Periodicals postage paid at New York, NY and additional mailing offices. Subscription price per year is $313.00 (US individuals), $633.00 (US institutions), $100.00 (US students), $366.00 (Canadian individuals), $833.00 (Canadian institutions), $100.00 (Canadian students), $429.00 (foreign individuals), $833.00 (foreign institutions), and $210.00 (foreign students). Foreign air speed delivery is included in all *Clinics* subscription prices. All prices are subject to change without notice. **POSTMASTER:** Send address changes to *Physical Medicine and Rehabilitation Clinics of North America*, Customer Service Office: Elsevier Health Sciences Division, Subscription Customer Service, 3251 Riverport Lane, Maryland Heights, MO 63043. **Customer Service: 1-800-654-2452 (US). From outside of the United States, call 314-447-8871. Fax: 314-447-8029. E-mail: JournalsCustomer Service-usa@elsevier.com (for print support); JournalsOnlineSupport-usa@elsevier.com (for online support).**

Physical Medicine and Rehabilitation Clinics of North America is indexed in *Excerpta Medica, MEDLINE/ PubMed (Index Medicus), Cinahl, and Cumulative Index to Nursing and Allied Health Literature.*

Contributors

CONSULTING EDITOR

SANTOS F. MARTINEZ, MD, MS
Diplomate of the American Academy of Physical Medicine and Rehabilitation, Certificate of Added Qualification Sports Medicine, Assistant Professor, Department of Orthopaedics, Campbell Clinic Orthopaedics, University of Tennessee, Memphis, Tennessee

EDITORS

STEVEN STANOS, DO
Director, Swedish Health System Pain Medicine and Services, Medical Director, Swedish Pain Services, Seattle, Washington

JAMES R. BABINGTON, MD
Staff Physician, Swedish Pain Services, Swedish Health System, Seattle, Washington, Swedish Pain Services, Swedish Medical Center, Edmonds, Washington

AUTHORS

TIMOTHY J. ATKINSON, PharmD, BCPS, CPE
Clinical Pharmacy Specialist, Pain Management, Director, PGY2 Pain Management and Palliative Care Pharmacy Residency, VA Tennessee Valley Healthcare System, Murfreesboro, Tennessee

JAMES R. BABINGTON, MD
Staff Physician, Swedish Pain Services, Swedish Health System, Seattle, Washington; Swedish Pain Services, Swedish Medical Center, Edmonds, Washington

WILSON J. CHANG, MD, MPH
Swedish Pain Services, Swedish Health System, Seattle, Washington

LINA FINE, MD, MPhil
Swedish Sleep Medicine, Swedish Medical Center, Seattle, Washington

ANDREW FRIEDMAN, MD
Section Head, Physical Medicine and Rehabilitation, Virginia Mason Medical Center, Clinical Assistant Profession, University of Washington, Seattle, Washington

JEFFREY FUDIN, BS, PharmD, FASHP, FCCP, FFSMB
Clinical Pharmacy Specialist, Pain Management, Director, PGY2 Pain Management and Palliative Care Pharmacy Residency, Albany Stratton VA Medical Center, Adjunct Associate Professor, Albany College of Pharmacy and Health Sciences, Albany, New York; CEO, Remitigate LLC, Delmar, New York

Topical Analgesics   233

Steven Stanos

> Topical analgesics are a growing area of clinical interest, given improvements in formulation drug delivery and local delivery of medicine, limiting risk for potential adverse systemic effects. Topical analgesics include medications for acute and chronic pain, such as musculoskeletal pain disorders, including sprains and strains; neuropathic pain; and muscle pain related to trauma. This review covers an update on formulations for acute and chronic pain, a discussion on advancements in drug delivery, and an update on recent treatment guidelines related to topical medications for osteoarthritis and neuropathic pain conditions.

Muscle Relaxants for Acute and Chronic Pain   245

Wilson J. Chang

> Utilization of muscle relaxants varies for treatment of acute and chronic pain. This article provides an overview of the different types muscles relaxants and their adverse effects. Appropriate medication selection based on clinical indications is also examined.

Pharmacologic Approach to Insomnia   255

Lina Fine

> Sleep management is essential to effective treatment of pain symptoms. Identification of the precise nature of sleep complaint, awareness of patient's age and co-morbid conditions and choice of the hypnotic medication class can help guide treatment approach. In addition to benzodiazepine and non-benzodiazepine medications acting at the GABA receptor, novel approaches, including orexin receptor agonists, may be safer and more promising pharmacologic approaches. Pharmacologic interventions, when used cautiously for a limited period of time and in complement with behavioral and cognitive approaches, can serve to improve sleep quality and significantly help in management of pain.

Opioid Management: Initiating, Monitoring, and Tapering   265

W. Michael Hooten

> Numerous guidelines targeting safe use of opioids for chronic pain have been published but substantial challenges persist in clinical application of best practice recommendations. This article describes a pragmatic approach to clinical care of adults with chronic pain receiving long-term opioid therapy. Three components of care are emphasized: (1) medical and mental health assessment before initiating opioid therapy, (2) clinical surveillance during the course of long-term opioid therapy, and (3) clinical considerations and strategies governing opioid tapering. A pressing need exists for ongoing research to further clarify the optimal role that long-term opioid therapy has in treatment of chronic pain.

Ethics and Regulation of Opioid Prescriptions for Management of Pain: The Washington State Experience   279

James R. Babington and Micah Matthews

> Painful conditions affect a significant population in the United States. As the scientific understanding of the benefits and harms of opioid therapy

has evolved, so too has the application of prescription opioid therapy for the treatment of pain. The rapid increase in the use of prescription and illicit opioids over the past decade has contributed to a public health crisis commonly referred to as the "opioid crisis." In this article, the ethical approaches to treating patients with opioid pharmaceuticals as well as the development of regulation of opioid therapy in Washington State are reviewed.

Opioids: Pharmacology, Physiology, and Clinical Implications in Pain Medicine   **289**

Andrew Friedman and Lorifel Nabong

Opioid receptors and opioid agonists are widespread throughout nature. Endogenous opioids mediate complex functions in animals and in humans. The opioid system in humans plays a central role in pain control and is a key mediator of hedonic homeostasis, mood, and well-being. This system also regulates responses to stress and several peripheral physiologic functions, including respiratory, gastrointestinal, endocrine, and immune systems. This article provides an overview of the basic physiology of opioids, reviews opioid pharmacology, and attempts to address several issues of current importance in the management of patients with established long-term opioid therapy.

PHYSICAL MEDICINE AND REHABILITATION CLINICS OF NORTH AMERICA

FORTHCOMING ISSUES

August 2020
Spinal Cord Injury
John L. Lin, *Editor*

November 2020
Integrative Medicine and Rehabilitation
Blessen C. Eapen and David Cifu, *Editors*

RECENT ISSUES

February 2020
Cerebral Palsy
Aloysia Leisanne Schwabe, *Editor*

November 2019
Rehabilitation in Developing Countries
Joseph P. Jacob, *Editor*

August 2019
Medical Impairment, Disability Evaluation and Associated Medicolegal Issues
Robert D. Rondinelli and Marjorie Eskay-Auerbach, *Editors*

SERIES OF RELATED INTEREST

Orthopedic Clinics
Clinics in Sports Medicine

VISIT THE CLINICS ONLINE!
Access your subscription at:
www.theclinics.com

Foreword
Resetting Pain Management Strategies

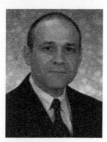

Santos F. Martinez, MD, MS
Consulting Editor

The field of pain management continues to be quite challenging as both patients and physicians adapt to ever-changing strategies. What may have been the standard of treatment just a few years ago now is found to be unacceptable especially with pharmacologic support. The medical field was encouraged to be sensitive to the pharmacologic management and support of this patient population with an array of innovative variations and methods. Standard intermittent administration of medications turned into longer-acting agents, including implants. Pain clinics became the in thing whether they were more pharmacologically or procedurally oriented. Some physicians became overreliant on physician extenders for day to day clinical management, only seeing patients when a procedure was to be performed. The use of opiates became center stage with an opiate epidemic and public health emergency declared. The repercussions continue to be felt by many medical physicians trying to help this patient population.

This issue allows us to reassess our options for treating pain. As we were taught years ago, each case needs to be individualized, whether that is treating a malignant versus a nonmalignant source of pain, understanding psychosocial and possibly genetic contributors, and accessing other adjunctive resources for a team approach, which is inherent to Physical Medicine and Rehabilitation. The editor hopes that every

Phys Med Rehabil Clin N Am 31 (2020) ix–x
https://doi.org/10.1016/j.pmr.2020.03.002
1047-9651/20/© 2020 Published by Elsevier Inc.

physician who receives this issue will be able to find a valuable tool to incorporate into their practice.

Santos F. Martinez, MD, MS
Physical Medicine and Rehabilitation
Department of Orthopaedics
University of Tennessee School of Medicine
Memphis, TN 38104, USA

E-mail address:
smartinez@campbellclinic.com

Preface

Pharmacologic Support in Pain Management

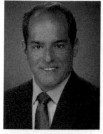 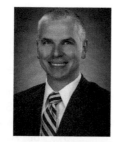

Steven Stanos, DO   James R. Babington, MD

Editors

The most effective pain management strategies rely on a comprehensive approach that addresses each aspect of the biopsychosocial model. At times patients warrant treatment with medication management, interventional pain management techniques, physical and occupational therapy, cognitive behavioral techniques, pain education, and interdisciplinary care. A critical factor in successful pharmacologic pain management is the ability to not only establish an accurate diagnosis but also tailor the treatment to address the underlying pathophysiologic and behavioral changes presenting as pain and pain-related suffering: a mechanistic approach that not only targets specific changes in the peripheral nervous system but also includes complex central changes at the spinal cord level and brain. Our aim in this issue of *Physical Medicine and Rehabilitation Clinics of North America* is to capture the current breadth of pharmacologic management of pain. In particular, we aim to highlight novel uses of pharmaceuticals and emerging therapeutics as well as review the more traditional pharmacologic approaches to pain management.

We review the use of buprenorphine in the treatment of chronic pain. The article skillfully helps the reader understand how to use this drug beyond its more common use as medication-assisted therapy for opioid use disorder. The review of emerging pharmacologic therapy for the treatment of pain introduces new therapeutic agents that provide promise in the future treatment of pain. We then review the more traditional pharmacologic agents, including nonsteroidal anti-inflammatory drugs, topical analgesics, and muscle relaxants. The article on pharmacotherapy for insomnia provides a primer on the broad group of agents used to help treat pain-related insomnia, a common and deleterious challenge to many patients suffering with persistent pain. The issue closes with a review of opioid monitoring, regulations, and the pharmacology of opioids. We hope that these articles in toto will help prescribers find a more balanced and safer approach to management of their patients with chronic pain.

Phys Med Rehabil Clin N Am 31 (2020) xi–xii
https://doi.org/10.1016/j.pmr.2020.03.001
1047-9651/20/© 2020 Published by Elsevier Inc.

pmr.theclinics.com

regarding its applicability in pain treatment. An example of this misrepresented pharmacology is the labeling of buprenorphine as a partial agonist of the mu opioid receptor. This classification has contributed to the myth of a ceiling effect on analgesia, born from findings of low intrinsic activity in test tube assays.[3] However, there is a key distinction between experimental intrinsic activity and clinical efficacy in people. Although a ceiling effect does exist with respect to buprenorphine's low potential for respiratory depression relative to other opioids, rendering it safer in clinical use, the analgesic activity of buprenorphine is dose-dependent without such a ceiling effect. Thus, it demonstrates a clinical profile more akin to a full agonist, as defined by production of full analgesia at less than 100% occupation of the mu opioid receptor.[4] In fact, buprenorphine exhibits effective analgesia at a relatively low receptor occupancy of 5% to 10%.[5] In terms of analgesic potency, buprenorphine is approximately 25 to 100 times more potent than morphine.[6]

Fig. 1 illustrates the relative therapeutic utility of buprenorphine and fentanyl, showing that within the same dose range, buprenorphine has a much greater likelihood of producing analgesia relative to risk of respiratory depression, whereas the opposite is true with fentanyl.

Another frequently misrepresented point regarding buprenorphine pharmacology relates to its high affinity for the mu opioid receptor,[7] and what effect this might have on the ability of other opioids to exert additional analgesia when used together with buprenorphine. Contrary to fears of blunted/absent effect at best and precipitated withdrawal or other acute reaction at worst, continuing use of buprenorphine as a baseline agent combined with another opioid after surgery or for treatment of acute pain of any cause has been shown in a multitude of studies to be safe and effective for analgesia.[8] Because therapeutic doses of buprenorphine do not occupy 100%

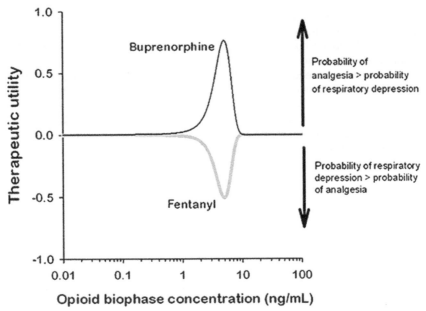

Fig. 1. Relative therapeutic utility of buprenorphine and fentanyl. (*Modified from* Yassen A, Olofsen E, Kan J, et al. Pharmacokinetic-pharmacodynamic modeling of the effectiveness and safety of buprenorphine and fentanyl in rats. Pharm Res. 2008; 25(1): 183-193; with permission.)

of available opioid receptors, unoccupied receptor availability can allow patients to achieve pain relief in varying degrees if a full opioid agonist is added to buprenorphine. Despite the scientific validity of continuing buprenorphine, some perioperative proto-cols continue to recommend cessation of buprenorphine prior to surgery because of fear of inadequate analgesia if it were to be continued. A recent systematic review of the literature acknowledged the lack of consistency on this point, but in its own conclusion strongly recommended continuation of buprenorphine throughout the peri-operative period in order to preserve stability for patients, many of whom have a his-tory of OUD as a cofactor being considered.[9] There does not appear to be any clinical advantage to stopping buprenorphine prior to surgery, while the harms may be signif-icant, especially in a patient susceptible to dangerous and/or non-medical opioid use.

Also related to the property of buprenorphine's strong affinity to the mu opioid re-ceptor, along with its slow association/dissociation kinetics, is the clinical question of reversibility of buprenorphine's agonist effects by the opioid receptor antagonist naloxone. Although lower doses of naloxone (0.5 mg) were shown to be ineffective, a 2 mg dose was shown to be sufficient to produce full reversal of respiratory depres-sion and restoration of normal minute ventilation.[10] Commonly used naloxone dosing, for example, in the commercially available intranasal spray formulation, is 4 mg, which is effective for reversal of buprenorphine. Of note, doses of naloxone above 5 mg are less effective in producing reversal of buprenorphine, as the naloxone:buprenorphine dose-response relationship is bell-shaped.[11]

There are 2 properties of buprenorphine that are not sources of clouded under-standing: reduced abuse liability compared with other opioids and reduced likelihood of inducing respiratory depression. Buprenorphine provides a primarily spinal site of mu opioid receptor agonist activity rather than direct activity at mu opioid receptors in the brain.[12] In this regard, it is different from fentanyl, morphine, and other more commonly used full agonist opioids, which appear to primarily affect brain mu opioid receptors. As opioid-induced respiratory depression is mediated by mu opioid recep-tors located in the brain stem, and the reinforcing effects of opioids are mediated through the brain's ventral tegmental area, nucleus accumbens, and prefrontal cortex (the mesolimbic system), it is therefore clinically significant that buprenorphine's activ-ity is directed primarily at the level of the spinal cord. This may further explain why a ceiling effect is displayed for respiratory depression but not for analgesia.[13]

One aspect of chronic pain that can be aggravated rather than relieved by chronic opioid therapy is the development of hyperalgesia.[14] Pain reduction by opioids largely results from activation of opioid receptors in the central nervous system (CNS) at both spinal and supraspinal levels, but opioids in general have a limited ability to prevent central sensitization of the pain pathways and subsequent hyperalgesia.[15] Mecha-nisms have been elucidated for development of hyperalgesia and its treatment, or antihyperalgesia, which are different from mechanisms for analgesia. This distinction was studied by Koppert and colleagues[16] in an investigation of the relative amounts of analgesia and antihyperalgesia from 3 different agents: alfentanil, a potent analogue of the opioid fentanyl; ketamine, an NMDA antagonist; and lidocaine, an anesthetic that acts via inhibition of sodium channels. It was found that of these 3 agents, while all temporarily reduced pain following administration, lidocaine produced the longest-lasting antihyperalgesic effect. Notably, buprenorphine blocks voltage-gated sodium channels via the local anesthetic binding site, which contributes to its pronounced antihyperalgesic effect[17] and is likely relevant in buprenorphine's efficacy in treating pain from neuropathic and chronic inflammatory conditions.

Another factor contributing to the antihyperalgesic effect of buprenorphine involves the role of the kappa opioid receptor. Although other opioids act as agonists of the kappa opioid receptor, thereby increasing the production of dynorphin, an endoge-nous opioid peptide known to contribute to hyperalgesia and antinociceptive toler-ance,[18] buprenorphine is the lone opioid that acts as an antagonist at the kappa opioid receptor. Therefore, buprenorphine use can counter one of the key mecha-nisms thought to be responsible for hyperalgesia and tolerance. This intrinsic antihy-peralgesic quality affords the practitioner the advantage of knowing that a patient maintained on buprenorphine who is experiencing inadequate pain control is not suffering from hyperalgesia induced from the buprenorphine itself, whereas long-term use of other opioids presents this clinical conundrum commonly.

Moreover, the role of dynorphin has been studied in the development of substance use disorders. Dynorphin systems may be recruited during the transition from episodic substance use to routine use and thus produce a negative emotional state in the absence of the drug, such as during withdrawal.[19] In blocking kappa opioid receptors and thereby removing the role of dynorphin in promoting a negative reinforcement loop for use of opioids, buprenorphine use for pain can be more reliably based on need for analgesia rather than avoidance of a negative emotional state.

In addition to its previously described effects on mu opioid receptors (agonist) and kappa opioid receptors (antagonist), buprenorphine displays weak agonist activity at delta opioid receptors and ORL-1 (nociceptin) receptors, although the contributions of these particular aspects of buprenorphine's opioid pharmacology to its overall anal-gesic effects are unclear. Of note, however, recent research in primates has high-lighted the potential utility of nociceptin production from a mu opioid receptor agonist in promoting analgesia with fewer opioid adverse effects.[20]

Compared with morphine and other opioids, buprenorphine has little or no immuno-suppressive effect[21] and appears less likely to suppress the gonadal axis or testos-terone levels.[22] Buprenorphine typically produces less slowing of intestinal motility and less constipation than morphine.[23] Buprenorphine neither blocks monoamine re-uptake nor is associated with the serotonin syndrome.[24]

FORMULATIONS OF BUPRENORPHINE USED FOR PAIN

The first buprenorphine formulation approved by the FDA for outpatient use for pain was the transdermal buprenorphine product in 2010, brand name Butrans. Although sublingual buprenorphine was approved by the FDA in 2002, the indication was for OUD, not pain. It is, however, frequently used in the treatment of chronic pain and will be discussed. The transdermal formulation was studied over periods of 3.4 years in patients with cancer pain and 5.75 years in patients with noncancer pain and was found to be subjectively effective for pain in 90% of all subjects.[25] It was generally well-tolerated, with the most common systemic adverse effects being nausea and dizziness; most common local skin reactions were erythema and pruritis. Other studies have shown buprenorphine to be effective, well-tolerated, and safe for pa-tients with severe cancer pain.[26]

In a German study that surveyed 9489 patients with chronic noncancer pain who were treated with transdermal buprenorphine, 80% reported their pain control as good or very good at final assessment, compared with 6% at initial assessment prior to stabilization on buprenorphine. Fewer than 5% discontinued treatment because of inadequate pain control. The tolerability profile was better than typical for opioids. Importantly, there was no clinically relevant development of tolerance.[27]

The manufacturer recommends discontinuing all around-the-clock opioids at the initiation of transdermal buprenorphine, but it does allow the use of short-acting opi-oids during titration periods. For patients receiving 30 to 80 mg oral morphine equivalent daily dose (MEDD), it is recommended to taper the dose to no more than 30 mg MEDD to reduce the risk of opioid withdrawal and inadequate pain control upon conversion to transdermal buprenorphine.

The recommended initial dose selection is based on the MEDD that the patient is currently receiving, as those receiving less than 30 mg and 30 to 80 mg of MEDD should be initiated on the 5 μg/h and 10 μg/h patch, respectively. Of note, a patient can apply up to 2 patches simultaneously during dose titrations, but it is important to apply both patches at the same time at 2 separate, adjacent application sites.

Buprenorphine patches should be left on for 7 days prior to removal. The dose can be titrated to a maximum of 20 μg/h in the United States, but doses above this have been shown to cause QT prolongation. This recommendation is based on a study cited in the prescribing information, which states that the 10 μg/h dose resulted in no clinically meaningful effect on mean QTc, whereas a 40 μg/h dose (2 20 μg/h patches) resulted in a maximum mean QTc prolongation of 9.2 ms across the 13 assessment time points.[28] This amount of prolongation is well below the level generally considered to be of clinical concern, which is 20 to 60 ms, with serious concern reserved for greater than 60 ms.[29] Notably, the current dose limit for transdermal buprenorphine in the United Kingdom is 140 μg/h, or 3.36 mg/d. Clearly, the limited dosing of this buprenorphine formulation in the United States has impacted its clinical utility, particularly with respect to patients transitioning to buprenorphine from other opioids taken at higher doses, such as 80 MEDD or greater. In a therapeutic review of buprenorphine in the *Journal of Pain and Symptom Management* from 2013, the authors characterized the dose limit on transdermal buprenorphine in the United States based on QTc interval concerns as "excessively restrictive."[30]

Dose adjustments should not be made until at least 72 hours of use at the same strength, as it takes 72 hours to achieve steady state concentrations. Time to peak concentration and elimination half-life are 60 hours and 26 hours, respectively.

A second buprenorphine product FDA approved for ambulatory use for chronic pain was buccal buprenorphine, brand name Belbuca, in 2015. Dosing ranges from 75 to 900 μg twice daily, given on a scheduled basis for patients requiring daily round-the-clock analgesia. There are no particular unique adverse effects with this formulation compared with previously available buprenorphine products. Although full prescribing information does mention the potential of QTc prolongation, there are no absolute contraindications to use in patients with history of cardiac arrhythmia. Most common adverse events in trials were the same for both opioid-experienced and opioid-naïve patients, and these included nausea, constipation, vomiting, and headache.[31]

A recent review of available medical literature focusing on the safety and efficacy of transdermal and buccal buprenorphine for treatment of chronic pain examined 33 studies, 29 focusing on transdermal and 4 on buccal film. Each and every study demonstrated efficacy for pain relief, and of the 28 studies that also assessed safety, each concluded that buprenorphine was safe and generally well-tolerated.[32]

For patients who are considering transitioning to buprenorphine for pain but are physiologically dependent on high doses of opioids, such as greater than 90 mg MEDD, off-label use of the higher potency sublingual buprenorphine formulation may be clinically appropriate to consider. As noted previously, sublingual buprenorphine was approved by the FDA for the indication of treatment of OUD in 2002. Because of limitations placed on prescribers of this formulation upon initial approval, which persist today for treatment of OUD, it has remained an underutilized tool in the treatment of OUD in the ongoing national response to the opioid crisis. It is even less typically considered and employed as a treatment option in the context of chronic pain treatment, especially when the diagnosis of OUD is not applicable to the patient. However, the US Department of Health and Human Services, in its recently released guide for tapering opioids, specifically calls for a greater role in promoting buprenorphine as an alternative pain management option for patients "on high opioid dosages unable to taper despite worsening pain and/or functioning with opioids, whether or not OUD criteria are met."[33]

As noted previously, buprenorphine is the subject of persistent myths regarding its pharmacology and efficacy for pain in comparison to traditional opioids, and these myths are especially prevalent with regard to the sublingual formulation, at least in part because of its historical use in treatment of OUD. Although the efficacy of buprenorphine in general as an analgesic has been evaluated thoroughly and conclusively,[34] the question of sublingual buprenorphine's effectiveness for pain has not been studied as extensively. A systematic review by Cote and Montgomery[35] in 2014 specifically examined the sublingual buprenorphine formulation and identified only 10 trials with a total of 1190 patients for inclusion. They concluded that "all studies reported that sublingual buprenorphine demonstrated some effectiveness as a chronic pain analgesic." However, they added that "due to the paucity of high-quality trials, the current evidence is insufficient to determine the effectiveness of sublingual buprenorphine for the treatment of chronic pain." Thus, lack of clarity and consensus persist regarding sublingual buprenorphine's effectiveness for pain, not because the available evidence is mixed, but because it is not considered to be of sufficient quality.

As noted previously, buprenorphine is commonly reported to have a ceiling effect for analgesia despite pharmacologic evidence that this is not the case. Sublingual buprenorphine plasma levels are dose proportional from 1 to 32 mg; sublingual absorption is not limiting. Buprenorphine plasma half-life is longer with sublingual administration than parenteral administration, related to slow release from buccal fat, which may act as a local depot.[36] Sublingual buprenorphine is available in 2 mg and 8 mg tablets, in film combined with naloxone as an abuse deterrent in 2/0.5 mg, 4/1 mg, 8/2 mg, and 12/3 mg, and in a more recently available buprenorphine/naloxone tablet with greater sublingual buprenorphine bioavailability that was approved by the FDA in July 2013 for OUD maintenance therapy. The newer formulation, branded Zubsolv, claims 30% greater buprenorphine bioavailability per milligram of buprenorphine relative to the generic formulation.[37] The 5.7/1.4 mg dose (buprenorphine/naloxone) tablet produces buprenorphine levels similar to the generic 8/2 mg tablet dose, and dissolves at a faster rate, while the sublingual film dissolves even faster than the newer buprenorphine/naloxone tablets (173 s on average, vs 242 s).[38]

PRACTICAL LIMITATIONS ON USE OF BUPRENORPHINE FOR PAIN

Prescribers who explicitly use sublingual buprenorphine for withdrawal management and maintenance therapy for OUD must register with the Center for Substance Abuse Treatment of the Substance Abuse and Mental Health Services Administration and undergo special training for certification and Drug Enforcement Agency (DEA) licensing. However, the FDA permits the use of sublingual buprenorphine as an off-label analgesic, despite common perception otherwise. The requirements for use of sublingual buprenorphine for pain involve only registering with the DEA as a prescriber of schedule III controlled medications. Training and registration as a prescriber for maintenance therapy of OUD are not required. However, it is important that prescribers using sublingual buprenorphine as an analgesic note on their prescriptions that it is explicitly being used for pain; otherwise pharmacies will not fill the prescription if the prescriber is not registered with the DEA for treatment of OUD. Some insurance companies attempt to limit sublingual buprenorphine to treatment of OUD only, restricting the potential use of this formulation in the treatment of pain. These unfortunate nonscientific obstacles to use of sublingual buprenorphine for pain have led to an ongoing underutilization of a potentially safe, effective, and sustainable management option for patients on chronic opioid therapy who do not meet criteria for OUD but may be experiencing other unintended negative consequences of high-dose opioid use, such as development of tolerance and hyperalgesia, and/or impairments in mood, cognition, sleep, and other aspects of functioning.

Another clinical obstacle to use of sublingual buprenorphine, whether for pain or treatment of OUD, is the necessity to introduce it when all or most opioid receptors are unoccupied, which in practice means the early phase of opioid withdrawal. If sublingual buprenorphine, which as noted previously has a high affinity for opioid receptors, is initiated while another opioid is still actively occupying a significant number of opioid receptors, the addition of buprenorphine can cause an abrupt displacement of the other opioid from its receptors, causing a precipitated withdrawal syndrome that tends to be clinically severe, although not typically life threatening. In order to avoid this outcome, patients being transitioned to sublingual buprenorphine must go through a washout period, allowing for the gradual onset of early withdrawal from the opioid being stopped, so that buprenorphine can be initiated ideally in an opioid-free receptor mileu.[39] For most short-acting opioids, 12 hours would be a sufficient window; for most extended-release formulations, 18 to 24 hours would be appropriate, with the exception of methadone or transdermal fentanyl, which may require 3 days or longer. There are microinduction techniques used where very low doses of buprenorphine can be introduced earlier in the withdrawal course, although these are more practical in an inpatient hospital setting where patients can be monitored carefully, and buprenorphine dosing can be titrated carefully under supervision.

Dosing of sublingual buprenorphine for pain is usually provided at least twice per day and up to every 6 hours based on the expected analgesic effect, in contrast to the once-daily dosing typically used for treatment of OUD, owing to buprenorphine's very long half-life, which is estimated at 20 to 73 hours. Stable levels do typically contribute to an even distribution of pain control through the 24-hour cycle. Onset of effect is 30 to 60 minutes following dosing, with peak at 1 to 4 hours. Elimination is primarily via stool, although 10% to 30% is excreted in urine as conjugated forms of buprenorphine and its metabolite norbuprenorphine (approximately 10%). Buprenorphine is considered a preferred opioid option for patients with either renal or hepatic disease.[40]

With a potential role to play in addressing the twin public health challenges of chronic pain and OUD treatment in the era of the opioid crisis, it could be instructive to examine recent trends in use of sublingual buprenorphine by clinicians specializing in pain medicine. One now potentially outdated study aimed to examine the extent to which pain specialists prescribe sublingual buprenorphine for chronic pain, along with associated clinician attitudes and behaviors.[41] Among a host of findings, it was noted that of the 230 clinicians surveyed (small sample size) in 2010 (likely not representative of current prescriber base, and performed before the availability of transdermal buprenorphine), 19.7% of them prescribed sublingual buprenorphine for pain. Of those, 64% had the DEA waiver to prescribe it for OUD. Sixty-five percent reported that switching to sublingual buprenorphine from another opioid was their greatest clinical challenge in using the medication.

In order to deter abuse of sublingual buprenorphine, a combination with the opioid receptor antagonist naloxone has been marketed since FDA approval in 2002. Naloxone has poor sublingual bioavailability (approximately 3%) so therefore is not clinically significant when used via this route; when used parenterally by an individual who has crushed tablets or melted down film, however, naloxone has good bioavailability, and its effect predominates and can precipitate an acute opioid withdrawal syndrome. The role of naloxone in the combination sublingual products has added to confusion over the pharmacology and clinical utility of buprenorphine among not only the lay public but also many clinicians who have only limited depth of understanding of buprenorphine's complex and unique pharmacology.[42]

SUMMARY

Buprenorphine has retained an air of mystery as an analgesic despite long-available pharmacologic data and clinical research that make clear its effectiveness for chronic pain in a broad spectrum of conditions. In addition, its safety advantages are well-known, along with its relative lack of psychomimetic effects in comparison to other opioids, which led to its use in the treatment of OUD. Its pronounced antihyperalgesic effect is a compelling pharmacologic attribute that makes it particularly attractive as an option for patients habituated to long-term, high-dose opioids who may be experiencing hyperalgesia but have not been educated regarding this phenomenon by their physicians, nor of the potential for buprenorphine to resolve it. As the number of elderly individuals with chronic pain increases in the United States, buprenorphine's superior safety profile and relative minimum of drug-drug interactions will make it particularly attractive in this population. Further curtailing comfort in the use of buprenorphine for pain is the specter of the DEA waiver requirement for use of the sublingual formulation in the treatment of OUD, and the common misconception that the waiver is required to prescribe sublingual buprenorphine for pain. The presence or absence of naloxone in combination with sublingual buprenorphine has provided additional nuance to an already pharmacologically complex opioid, further fueling perception of clinical management challenges from the perspective of both patients and care providers. For these reasons, some prescribers of traditional opioids, even pain specialists, unfortunately may consider use of buprenorphine to be outside their scope of practice. These limitations on potential and actual utilization are generally based on factors other than accurate understanding of the pharmacology, safety, and effectiveness of buprenorphine. In the current climate, in which the role of opioids in the treatment of chronic pain is undergoing an evolutionary reassessment, it is critical that high-quality studies emerge to dispel myths and underscore the known advantages and possibilities of buprenorphine. Until then, there is more than enough data to compel providers to consider buprenorphine as a first-line opioid choice for patients with chronic pain who require a long-acting opioid analgesic.

DISCLOSURE

No disclosures.

REFERENCES

1. Cowan A, Lewis JW, Macfarlane IR. Agonist and antagonist properties of buprenorphine, a new antinociceptive agent. Br J Pharmacol 1977;60(4):537–45.
2. Jasinki DR, Pevnick JS, Griffith JD. Human pharmacology and abuse potential of the analgesic buprenorphine: a potential agent for treating narcotic addiction. Arch Gen Psychiatry 1978;35(4):501–16.
3. Traynor JR. G-protein coupling and efficacy of μ-opioid agonists: relationship to behavioral efficacy. Rev Analg 2004;8:11–22.

4. Greenwald MK, Comer SD, Fiellin DA. Buprenorphine maintenance and *mu*-opioid receptor availability in the treatment of opioid use disorder: implications for clinical use and policy. Drug Alcohol Depend 2014;0:1–11.
5. Heit HA, Gourlay DL. Buprenorphine: new tricks with an old molecule for pain management. Clin J Pain 2008;24(2):93–7.
6. Khanna IK, Pillarisetti S. Buprenorphine - an attractive opioid with underutilized potential in treatment of chronic pain. J Pain Res 2015;8:859–70.
7. Huang P, Kehner GB, Cowan A, et al. Comparison of pharmacological activities of buprenorphine and norbuprenorphine: norbuprenorphine is a potent opioid agonist. J Pharmacol Exp Ther 2001;297:688–95.
8. Oifa S, Sydoruk T, White I, et al. Effects of intravenous patient-controlled analgesia with buprenorphine and morphine alone and in combination during the first 12 postoperative hours: a randomized, double-blind, four-arm trial in adults undergoing abdominal surgery. Clin Ther 2009;31(3):527–41.
9. Ward EN, Quaye AN-A, Willens TE. Opioid use disorders: perioperative management of a special population. Anesth Analg 2018;127(2):539–47.
10. Dahan A, Yassen A, Bijl H, et al. Buprenorphine induces ceiling in respiratory depression but not in analgesia. Br J Anaesth 2006;96:627–32.
11. Van Dorp E, Yassen A, Sarton E, et al. Naloxone reversal of of buprenorphine-induced respiratory depression. Anesthesiology 2006;105:51–7.
12. Ding Z, Raffa RB. Identification of an additional supraspinal component to the analgesic mechanism of action of buprenorphine. Br J Pharmacol 2009;157:831–43.
13. Dahan A. Opioid-induced respiratory effects: new data on buprenorphine. Palliat Med 2006;20:53–8.
14. Celerier E, Rivat C, Jun Y, et al. Long-lasting hyperalgesia induced by fentanyl in rats: preventative effect of ketamine. Anesthesiology 2000;92:465–72.
15. Moiniche S, Kehlet H, Dahl JB. A qualitative and quantitative systematic review of preemptive analgesia for postoperative pain relief. Anesthesiology 2002;96:725–41.
16. Koppert W, Dern S, Sittl R, et al. A new model of electrically evoked pain and hyperalgesia in human skin. Anesthesiology 2001;95:395–402.
17. Leffler A, Frank G, Kistner K, et al. Local anesthetic-like inhibition of voltage-gated Na(+) channels by the partial mu opioid receptor agonist buprenorphine. Anesthesiology 2012;116(6):1335–46.
18. Vanderrah TW, Gardell LR, Burgess SE, et al. Dynorphin promotes abnormal pain and spinal opioid antinociceptive tolerance. J Neurosci 2000;20:7074–9.
19. Walker BM, Valdez GR, McLaughlin JP, et al. Targerting dynorphin/kappa opioid receptor systems to treat alcohol abuse and dependence. Alcohol 2012;46(4):359–70.
20. Ding H, Kiguchi N, Yasuda D, et al. A bifunctional nociceptin and mu opioid receptor agonist is analgesic without opioid side effects in nonhuman primates. Sci Transl Med 2018;10(456):eaar3483.
21. Sacerdote P. Opioids and the immune system. Palliat Med 2006;20:S9–15.
22. Hallinan R, Byrne A, Agho K, et al. Hypogonadism in men receiving methadone and buprenorphine maintenance treatment. Int J Androl 2007;32:131–9.
23. Pace MC, Passavanti MB, Grella E, et al. Buprenorphine in long-term control of chronic pain in cancer patients. Front Biosci 2007;12:1291–9.
24. Rickli A, Liakoni E, Hoener MC, et al. Opioid-induced inhibition of the human 5-HT and noradrenaline transporters in vitro: link to clinical reports of serotonin syndrome. Br J Pharmacol 2018;175(3):532–43.

25. Likar R, Kayser H, Sittl R. Long-term management of chronic pain with transdermal buprenorphine: a multi-center, open-label, follow-up study in patients from three short-term clinical trials. Clin Ther 2006;28:943–52.

26. Poulain P, Denier W, Douma J, et al. Efficacy and safety of transdermal buprenorphine: a randomized, placebo-controlled trial in 289 patients with severe cancer pain. J Pain Symptom Manage 2008;36:117–25.

27. Greissinger N, Sittl R, Likar R. Transdermal buprenorphine in clinical practice: a post-marketing surveillance study in 13,179 patients. Curr Med Res Opin 2005; 21:1147–56.

28. Purdue Pharma LP. Butrans full prescribing information. Stanford (CT): USFDA; 2010.

29. Twycross R, Wilcock A. Prolongation of the QT interval in palliative care. Palliative care formulary. 4th edition 2011.

30. Foster B, Twycross R, Mihalyo M, et al. Buprenorphine. J Pain Symptom Manage 2013;45(5):939–49.

31. Endo Pharmaceuticals. Belbuca full prescribing information. Malvern (PA): USFDA; 2015.

32. Pergolizzi JV Jr, Raffa RB. Safety and efficacy of the unique opioid buprenorphine for the treatment of chronic pain. J Pain Res 2019;12:3299–317.

33. Dowell D, Jones C, Compton W, et al. HHS guide for clinicians on the appropriate dosage reduction or discontinuation of long-term opioid analgesics. Available at: HHS.gov. Accessed October, 2019.

34. Raffa RB, Haidery M, Huang HM, et al. The clinical analgesic efficacy of buprenorphine. J Clin Pharm Ther 2014;39(6):577–83.

35. Cote J, Montgomery L. Sublingual buprenorphine as an analgesic in chronic pain: a systematic review. Pain Med 2014;15(7):1171–8.

36. Kuhlman JJ, Lalani S, Magluilo J Jr, et al. Human pharmacokinetics of intravenous, sublingual, and buccal buprenorphine. J Anal Toxicol 1996;20(6):369–78.

37. Orexo US. Inc. Zubsolv full prescribing information. Morristown (NJ): USFDA; 2013.

38. Gunderson E, Sumner M. Efficacy of buprenorphine/naloxone rapidly dissolving sublingual tablets (BNX-RDT) after switching from BNX sublingual film. J Addict Med 2016;10(2):122–8.

39. Manhapra A, Arias A, Ballantyne JC. The conundrum of opioid tapering in long-term opioid therapy for chroniuc pain: a commentary. Subst Abus 2018;39(2): 152–61.

40. Lufty K, Cowan A. Buprenorphine: a unique drug with complex pharmacology. Curr Neuropharmacol 2004;2(4):395–402.

41. Rosen K, Gutierrez A, Haller D, et al. Sublingual buprenorphine for chronic pain: a survey of clinician prescribing practices. Clin J Pain 2014;30(4):295–300.

42. Mendelsohn J, Jones RT. Clinical and pharmacological evaluation of buprenorphine and naloxone combinations: why the 4:1 ratio for treatment? Drug Alcohol Depend 2003;70(2 Suppl):S29–37.

Evolving Pharmacotherapies for Pain: Drug Development

Rohit Nalamasu, DO[a],*, Srinivas Nalamachu, MD[b]

KEYWORDS

- Pain pharmacotherapy • Chronic pain • Novel pain management
- Nerve growth factors • Nav 1.7 • Tenazumab
- Calcitonin gene–related peptide (CGRP) • Condoliase

KEY POINTS

- Anti-nerve growth factor antibodies are in late-stage clinical development for the treatment of chronic pain secondary to osteoarthritis, chronic low back pain, and potentially cancer-related pain.
- Nav1.7, Nav1.8, and Nav1.9 are voltage-gated sodium channels that have been the newly studied analgesic targets, linked with the peripheral nervous system, and are associated with pain disorders of monogenic origin.
- Various N-methyl-D-aspartate receptor modulators are currently being evaluated for various neurologic disorders including centrally mediated pain.
- NKTR-181 is a long-acting full mu-agonist that provides pain relief with limited euphoric effects, designed to lead to less addiction potential.
- Calcitonin gene–related peptides are thought to have an important role in migraine processing. The receptors are located at spots involved in migraine pathogenesis and increase during migraines and fall after treatment.

Chronic pain epidemic is one of the most discussed and pressing public health crises facing the United States today. As society becomes increasingly focused on drug misuse, abuse, opioid addiction, and overdose deaths, clinicians treating those patients with chronic pain struggle with increased scrutiny. Currently, more than 100 million Americans suffer from chronic pain,[1] with chronic pain being among the most prevalent conditions and the leading cause of disability.[2] The Centers for Disease Control and Prevention (CDC) in 2016 noted an estimated 20.4% of US adults have chronic pain with 8% of the same population suffering from high-impact chronic pain.[3] These diagnoses have been linked to significant limitations in mobility and activities of daily living, reduced quality of life, increased opioid dependence, anxiety and depression, as well as poor perceived health. Chronic pain disproportionally affects

[a] Physical Medicine and Rehabilitation, University of Nebraska, 986155 Nebraska Medical Center, Omaha, NE 68198-6155, USA; [b] Mid-America Poly Clinic, 7100 College Boulevard, Overland Park, KS 66210, USA
* Corresponding author.
E-mail address: rohit.nalamasu@unmc.edu

Phys Med Rehabil Clin N Am 31 (2020) 205–217
https://doi.org/10.1016/j.pmr.2020.01.001

women, older adults, adults living in poverty, unemployed but previously employed adults, rural-living adults, and adults with public health insurance (both Medicare and Medicaid). The CDC study also noted a higher, but statistically insignificant number of high-impact chronic pain in Caucasian adults compared with other ethnic groups and veterans compared with nonveterans, accommodating for differences in age and other demographics. As our population is aging and life expectancy is improving with increased access to health care and better-quality health care, we expect to see an increase in number of people suffering from chronic pain.

The current opioid crisis is a multifactorial public health crisis affecting America and the western world. According to the former surgeon general, more than 2.5 million people are addicted to opioid medications including both prescription drugs as well as illicit substances such as heroin and fentanyl, with another 12 misusing them. This results in 90 opioid overdose deaths in the United States alone.[4] An additional 11 million older than the age of 12 years have been shown to misuse these medications in 2017.[5] Heroin deaths have quadrupled from 2010 to 2016 reaching nearly 15,500 deaths annually with nearly a million users in 2016. Nonmedical users of opioid medications were 40 times more likely to abuse heroin. Fentanyl is 50 times more potent than heroin and 100 times more potent than morphine and has contributed to 20,000 overdose deaths in 2016, twice more than 2015. This increase is primarily attributed to the increase of illicit fentanyl.[6]

As the presence of the current opioid crisis and chronic pain epidemics demonstrate, there is a need for novel therapies to better manage chronic pain, as well as improved formulations of current medications, to mitigate risk associated with misuse and abuse.

Multiple abuse-deterrent opioid formulations (ADFs) of various known molecular entities have been developed, which have shown to provide the intended pain relief while limiting the potential for misuse and abuse. Despite current evidence showing tamper resistance in the clinical trial setting, there is insufficient evidence showing that ADFs have had a significant effect on opioid overdose and addiction in the real world.[7] ADFs can potentially tackle multiple avenues of abuse potential including the issues of alternative routes of administration that abusers use to provide faster drug delivery and onset. Few novel ADF technologies may be of worth reviewing by the practitioner.

This article focuses primarily on new molecular entities in development targeting various chronic pain receptors and new delivery technologies. Several biochemical mediators such as prostaglandins, cytokines, growth factors (ie, nerve growth factor [NGF], brain-derived neurotrophic factor), chemokines, and several neuropeptides (ie, substance P, calcitonin gene–related peptide [CGRP]) are involved in the current understanding of the chronic pain pathway. Chronic pain (greater than 3 months) involves biochemical changes in the nervous system. Increased levels of biochemical mediators lead to increased numbers of pain signals through the peripheral nervous system, known as peripheral sensitization. Peripheral sensitization can in turn lead to central sensitization, the alteration of central nervous system (CNS) neurons, leading to continuous high pain reactivity, and a heightened perception of pain. **Fig. 1** highlights the current understanding of the chronic pain pathway and the various receptors involved.

CAPSAICIN

Capsaicin is an agonist for the neural transient receptor potential cation channel subfamily V member 1 (TRPV-1). TRPV1 opens with heat, acid, and certain fatty acid exposure and has pronociceptive effects.[8] Capsaicin targets TRPV1 receptor to selectively inactivate local pain fibers to provide pain relief.

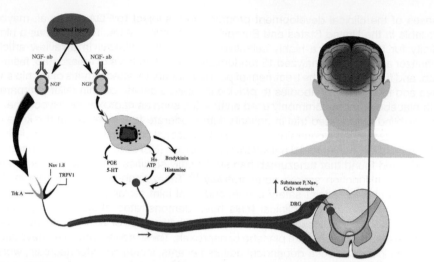

Fig. 1. Different receptors and regulatory mechanisms involved in chronic pain.

Transdermal Capsaicin

Qutenza is an 8% high-concentration capsaicin transdermal patch indicated in the European Union for treatment of peripheral neuropathic pain in adults and indicated by the Food and Drug Administration (FDA) for the treatment of pain associated with postherpetic neuralgia in the United States. High-concentration topical capsaicin was also found to treat peripheral neuropathic conditions such as human immunodeficiency virus neuropathy and diabetic neuropathy minimally better than low-concentration topical capsaicin.[9] In patients who had significant pain relief, low-dose capsaicin also showed improvement of secondary endpoints such as sleep, fatigue, depression, and quality of life compared with low-dose capsaicin. Insufficient data exist to show meaningful impact of low-concentration capsaicin cream in neuropathic pain treatment compared with placebo.[10] Currently there is a clinical trial assessing the efficacy of the Qutenza (capsaicin) patch in patients with cancer with neuropathic pain.

Intraarticular Capsaicin

An ultra-pure synthetic form of intraarticular trans-capsaicin has been shown to have dose-dependent improvement in pain secondary to osteoarthritis of the knee in a randomized double-blind study.[11] Clinical trial data suggest potential pain relief with intraarticular trans-capsaicin for up to 6 months until regeneration of local pain fibers.[12]

MONOCLONAL ANTIBODIES

Anti-NGF antibodies are monoclonal antibodies that are in late-stage clinical development for the treatment of chronic pain secondary to osteoarthritis, chronic low back pain, and potentially cancer-related pain. Antagonism of NGF is known to cause analgesia due to its involvement in chronic pain. Nerve growth factor increases nociceptive sensitization, and inflammation sites have been shown to have increased expression of nerve growth factor protein.[13,14]

Tanezumab

Tanezumab is the first of its kind in this class of drugs to have received fast track designation by the FDA for the treatment of chronic pain. Tenazumab is in the late phases of the clinical development program and, subject to FDA approval, maybe available in the United States and Europe in the coming years. The drug has a high affinity for NGF and is a highly selective monoclonal antibody. In a review article Schnitzer and Marks[15] analyzed 13 randomized controlled trials of tenazumab, fasinumab, and fulranumab in the treatment of pain secondary to osteoarthritis of the hip and knee and found NGF antibodies to provide increased benefit of pain relief compared with placebo or more commonly used analgesics such as naproxen or oxycodone. A double-blind randomized trial in patients with moderate-to-severe OA of the knee or hip who failed or had a contraindication to conventional analgesic treatment (including acetaminophen, nonsteroidal antiinflammatory drugs [NSAIDs], and either tramadol or opioids) and found that tanezumab had statistically significant improvements in pain and physical function scores comparatively.[16] Tanezumab-treated patients in the study also had more joint safety events and total joint replacements. Higher doses of tenazumab in previous clinical trials have demonstrated statistically significant pain relief in the chronic low back pain population with doses of 10 mg or 20 mg doses every 8 weeks compared with placebo or naproxen. These doses, however, have seen greater incidence of dose-dependent adverse events, including osteonecrosis, worsening osteoarthritis, and total joint replacements.[17]

Fasinumab and Fulranumab

Fasinumab is another NGF antibody that has been studied primarily in hip/knee OA and chronic low back pain. A recent 2019 phase IIb/III trial studying trial doses of 1 mg, 3 mg, 6 mg, and 9 mg showed improvements in hip and knee osteoarthritis pain and function, when compared with placebo, in patients who had inadequate pain relief or intolerance to conventional analgesic therapy including acetaminophen, greater than one oral NSAID, and greater than one opioid (or unwillingness to use opioids). The trial revealed increased dose-dependent adverse effects of arthropathy with one case of destructive arthropathy in a 6-mg dose patient.[18] Clinical development program for regulatory approval is currently in progress.

A clinical development program for a third drug in this class, fulranumab, had early clinical trials, but development has been halted by the sponsor.

SODIUM CHANNEL BLOCKERS

Nav1.7, Nav1.8, and Nav1.9 are voltage-gated sodium channels that have been the newly studied analgesic targets. These channels have been linked with the peripheral nervous system more than CNS and are associated with pain disorders of monogenic origin (**Fig. 2**).

Nav1.7

Of these, Nav1.7 is the most studied. Animal studies have indicated a role of Nav1.7 in acquired channelopathies, as it is upregulated in peripheral tissue inflammation and can lead to neuronal hyperexcitability. Studies done have shown that Nav1.7 knockout results in upregulation of enkephalins, suggesting a role in endogenous opioid signaling.[19]

The medications were studied after finding an apparent pain-free child in Pakistan who was damaging himself for tourists by sticking knives through his arms and walking across coals. A Cambridge-led team identified mutations in the SCN9A (on chromosome 2q31–32) gene that encodes Nav1.7, leading to this condition known as congenital insensitivity to pain.[20] SCN9A mutations have been linked to other inherited pain syndromes as well via gain-of-function mutations, such as inherited

Sodium Channel Isoforms

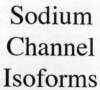

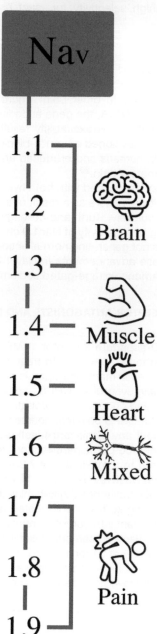

Fig. 2. Sodium channel isoforms.

erythromelalgia and paroxysmal extreme pain disorder, which suggests that Nav1.7 is involved in pain signaling. A Nav1.7 deletion study in mice indicated loss of acute and inflammatory pain with greater specificity for Nav1.7 over cardiac Nav1.5 but poor specificity compared with brain Nav 1.2 and Nav 1.6.[21] Early attempts at inhibiting the channel have been unsuccessful, as it has been difficult to block Nav1.7 alone and not structurally related ion channels, but some tarantula peptide-mimicking microproteins have shown high selectivity for Nav1.7 over Nav1.2 (80-fold) and Nav1.6 (20-fold).[22]

Nav1.8 and Nav1.9

Along with Nav1.7, Nav1.8 and Nav1.9 have also been studied as novel pain therapeutic receptors. The receptors are located predominantly in the peripheral nervous system and have been associated with other pain syndromes. Two gain-of-function mutations were discovered in SCN10A, the gene encoding Nav1.8. These mutations led to painful neuropathy via the hyperexcitability resulting from increased altered channel activity.[19] Researchers developed a Nav1.8-blocking compound that reduced neuronal excitability in vitro in humans and produced analgesia in rodent models of both neuropathic and inflammatory pain.[23]

Nav1.9 has conversely been associated with both hypersensitivity and insensitivity to painful stimuli. Hypersensitivity occurs as a result of a gain-of-function mutation in the SCN11A gene. Counterintuitively, Kurth and colleagues described a point mutation in SCN11A, with resulting hyperactivity of Nac1.9 channels leading to pain insensitivity. This is a result of cells not generating normal action potentials due to constant depolarization.[24] Despite these advancements in Nav 1.8 and Nav1.9, Nav1.7 continues to be the main target among voltage-gated sodium channels in pain analgesia.

N-METHYL-D-ASPARTATE RECEPTOR ANTAGONISTS AND MODULATORS
Ketamine

Ketamine is an N-methyl-D-aspartate receptor (NMDA) antagonist that is used frequently for sedation, anesthesia, as well as to treat acute and chronic pain. Ketamine infusions have been studied in many neuropathic pain conditions including fibromyalgia, complex regional pain syndrome (CRPS), spinal cord injury, phantom limb pain, postherpetic neuralgia, and oncogenic neuropathic pain.[25]

Ketamine infusion studies for CRPS pain management have shown initial pain relief that tapered off in time without any significant functional improvement. Sigtermans and colleagues[26] noted in their 60-participant randomized controlled trial trial, with a rate of 1.2 µg/kg/min titrated to a maximum of 7.2 µg/kg/min for 5 days, that the benefit was greatest in the first week and lasted for 11 weeks. Kiefer and colleagues[27] studied anesthetic dosages of intravenous (IV) ketamine (bolus 1.5 mg/kg followed by titration from 3 mg/kg/h to 7 mg/kg/h while intubated and ventilated for 5 days) in CPRS. In Kiefer's study CRPS went into complete remission at 1 month in all patients and at 6 months for 80% of patients. Mean pain relief in all patients in this open-label study was 93.5% at month, 89.4% at 3 months, and 79.3% at 6 months. In those participants with relapsing CRPS, significant pain relief was seen at 3 and 6 months. Quality of life, ketamine-associated movement disorder, and work ability improved in most of the patients at 3 and 6 months as well.

In a study of phantom limb pain, Eichenberger and colleagues studied calcitonin and ketamine in a double-blind, randomized control trial crossover study in which the treatment arms were calcitonin, ketamine, ketamine with calcitonin, or placebo. Patients in this trial were given 0.4 mg/kg over 1 hour of ketamine and found that ketamine with or without calcitonin resulted in significantly reduced pain intensity (50% and 60%) versus after calcitonin alone or placebo (10%) for 48 hours postinfusion.[28]

Although ketamine IV seems to have promising results, current data are limited by the small sample size, its randomized controlled trials, and its lack of consistency of variables such as dosing and length of treatment between studies.

Regarding topical ketamine, results have been mixed in the literature. One double-blind randomized controlled trial study comparing 1% ketamine, 2% amitriptyline, and a combination TID for 3 weeks showed a greater reduction of pain score (50%) in 10% of patients who received ketamine compared with placebo (18%).[29] Another study examined its use in 5 outpatient spinal cord injury patients, where participants were given 10% topical ketamine TID for 2 weeks, with resulting pain reduction from 14% to 63%.[30] A study of 5% topical ketamine cream applied for 1 month in patients with diabetic neuropathy was found to be no more effective at relieving than placebo.[31]

N-Methyl-D-Aspartate Receptor Modulators

Various NMDA modulators are currently being evaluated for various neurologic disorders including centrally mediated pain. NYX-2925 is an NMDA receptor modulator currently in phase 2 clinical development for treatment of chronic pain via central pain processing effects. Favorable safety and tolerability profiles seen on phase 1 and 2 testing has led to fast track designation from the FDA for neuropathic pain from diabetic peripheral neuropathy. Other NMDA modulators currently in development include NYX-783, being developed for the treatment of posttraumatic stress disorder, and NYX-458, being developed for the treatment of cognitive impairment associated with Parkinson disease.[32]

BUPRENORPHINE FORMULATIONS

Although buprenorphine has traditionally been used for the treatment of opioid addiction, low-dose buprenorphine has been shown to be helpful in the management of pain. The FDA has approved buprenorphine in 2 formulations for the treatment of chronic pain: Butrans patch and Belbuca sublingual formulation.

Transdermal Patch

The low molecular weight, potency, and lipophilic properties of buprenorphine make it an ideal candidate for transdermal delivery. BUTRANS (R) low-dose transdermal buprenorphine was found to be beneficial in the treatment of moderate-to-severe chronic pain in opioid-naïve patients without unanticipated safety findings using 7-day patches.[33] In the United States, BUTRANS (R) patch is available in 5, 7.5, 10, 15, and 20 mcg/h strengths with a q7 day dosing. Most common side effects were nausea, application site pruritus, headache, somnolence, dizziness, constipation, and application site erythema/rash/irritation. Abuse via snorting, swallowing, injecting, or chewing the buprenorphine from the transdermal system continues to be a concern.[34]

Sublingual Buprenorphine

Belbuca is a sublingual buprenorphine formulation whose efficacy has been evaluated in 3 12-week double-blind, placebo-controlled clinical trials in opioid-naïve and opioid-experienced patients with moderate-to-severe chronic low back pain. Two of the studies noted statistically significant efficacy differences between placebo and

Belbuca, and one study showed no statistically significant pain reduction. A higher proportion of Belbuca patients had a greater than 30% and 50% pain reduction compared with placebo in opioid-naïve patients and opioid-experienced patients in the studies.[35]

Formulations with Limited Euphoria

NKTR-181 is a long-acting full mu-agonist that provides pain relief with limited euphoric effects, designed to lead to less addiction potential. With the addition of a polyethylene glycol group, the drug has slower permeation through the blood brain barrier, with less euphoria as a result. The slower permeation also leads to longer-acting pain relief with a lengthened initiation of action. The medication is dosed q12 hours. Preclinical data from Nektar Therapeutics showed decreased rate of CNS entry through any route of administration. A phase-3 program compared BID dosing of 4 dosages (100 mg, 200 mg, 300 mg, 400 mg) of NKTR-181 with placebo in 600 opioid-naive patients with moderate-to-severe chronic low back pain and found that patients on average had greater than 65% pain reduction with a favorable safety profile. The medication had less drug-liking, drug high, and repeat drug scores compared with oxycodone, 40 mg and 60 mg, even when using a supratherapeutic dose of NKTR-181[36] in a 52-week-long safety study. NKTR-181 has not yet received FDA approval but has been granted fast-track designation for the treatment of moderate-to-severe chronic pain by the FDA.

Calcitonin Gene–Related Peptide Inhibitors and Modulators

CGRPs are thought to have an important role in migraine processing. The receptors are located at spots involved in migraine pathogenesis and increase during migraines and decrease after treatment. The peptide's release results in vasodilation and neurogenic inflammation. CGRP inhibitors and modulators aim to block or remove CGRP, which has been shown to terminate migraines acutely and also prevent them.[37]

CGRP antagonists with the "-gepant" distinction had its first proof in olcegepant, which had a clinical effect on humans in 2004 but was not brought to market due to inability to be orally administered. Telcagepant had a clinical effect in the past but had a hepatotoxic risk that stopped development.[38] Rimegepant, administered orally in 75 mg doses via an oral dissolving formulation, was found to be more effective than placebo with similar tolerability in migraine treatment in a randomized, double-blind phase III trial.[39] Ubrogepant, administered 25 mg, 50 mg, and 100 mg orally in randomized, double-blind, phase III trials noted significant 2-hour pain freedom and 2-hour absence of migrane-associated symptom for the 50-mg arm, with higher pain relief rates as well. In the clinical trials, no hepatotoxicity was noted with ubrogepant.[40,41] Both rimegepant and ubrogepant have been approved by the FDA for treatment of acute migraine.

Monoclonal antibodies to the CGRP erenumab was approved in May 2018 for migraine prevention and galcanezumab and fremanezumab approved in November 2018 also for migraine prevention. Erenumab is humanized immunoglobulin G2 monoclonal antibody administered monthly subcutaneously in doses of 70 mg and 140 mg that targets CRGP receptor. Clinical trials showed increasing numbers of participants getting greater than 50% reduction in monthly migraine days in those receiving erenumab compared with placebo without significant adverse effects.[37] Eptinezumab binds to α and β forms of the human CGRP ligand and administered intravenously every 12 weeks. Three completed phase III clinical trials (PROMISE I, PROMISE II, and PREVAIL) have yet to be published in peer-reviewed journals, but preliminary data from press releases indicate that the medication was efficacious in episodic and chronic migraine in phase 2 studies and episodic migraines in phase 3 studies.

Alpha-2 Antagonists

Tolperisone, a centrally acting muscle relaxant via alpha-2 antagonism used outside of the United States for treatment of elevated muscle tone, is primarily used in conditions associated with painful reflexic muscle spasms and lumbar pain, cervical and cervico-brachial syndrome, muscle trauma, sports injuries, and in spastic neurologic diseases such as multiple sclerosis. Unlike benzodiazepines, tolperisone is not associated with hepatotoxicity or drowsiness.[42,43] The mechanism of action is not fully understood, but its inhibitory actions on mono- and polysynaptic spinal reflexes and inhibitory actions on supraspinal descending pathways is considered the main method of action on spasms and spasticity. It also exhibits properties similar to local anesthetics such as lidocaine. It contains both sodium (on voltage-gated sodium channels) and calcium channel blocking both presynaptically and postsynaptically along with alpha antagonist (α1D and α2A) and muscarinic antagonist effects.[44] Most common side effects of the medication in published trials have been weakness (0.9%) and disorders of the digestive tract (0.7%).[45] These effects disappeared in trials where the medication was administered for more than several months.[46] Three placebo controlled double-blind trials accessed the use of tolperisone in the treatment of painful muscle spasms, all showing statistically significant effects with doses ranging from 300 mg to 900 mg a day.[47] The medication is absorbed easily and distributed widely, including to the CNS, and excreted via the kidneys. Analgesic effects, in particular, have been studied in mice where low-dose oral administration produced analgesia to heat.[48–50]

Mucopolysaccharidase

Condoliase (chondroitin sulfate ABC endolyase) is a pure mucopolysaccharidase derived from the gram-negative rod *Proteus vulgaris*. The drug has a high substrate specificity to glycosaminoglycans such as chondroitin sulfate and hyaluronic acid in the nucleus pulposis of the intervertebral disc. Previous drug in the same class, chymopapain, was approved by the FDA in 1982 for lumbar disc herniation treatment and had up to 80% symptom improvement in many studies but had a low substrate specificity. This, along with poor user training, resulted in anaphylactic reactions and significant neurologic complications such as paraplegia and transverse myelitis that resulted in the discontinuation of the product in 1999.

Condoliase was studied at 35 Japanese medical institutions in patients with clinically significant lumbar disc herniation, and the treatment arm of the study was compared with placebo up to 52 weeks after injection. The primary outcome was daily leg pain up to 13 weeks postinjection with secondary endpoints including back pain, oswestry disability index, neurologic examinations, short-form health survey, volumes of intervertebral disc and herniated masses on MRI, disc heights on radiograph, and lumbar surgery performed before week 52. In the study, Condoliase had statistically significant changes in symptoms, physical functions, and quality of life compared with placebo without tolerability issues.[51] It is approved for the treatment of lumbar disk herniation in Japan and is currently being studied in the United States.[52]

The novel pharmacotherapeutic options discussed in this article show significant promise for the future of chronic pain treatment and opioid alternatives. Some of these new therapies have the potential to be analgesics with proven efficacy and less addictive properties. As the authors continue to expand their research and development in the area, more novel pharmacotherapies are likely to be developed and will have a profound positive impact on the management of chronic pain. Better pain management education, along with more available options to the health care provider, will be a key component in addressing the epidemics of chronic pain and the opioid overdose crisis. The authors hope that this in-turn will continue to spur development of more novel chronic pain therapies.

DISCLOSURE

S. Nalamachu: Paid consultant/research investigator for Pfizer, Lilly, Neurana, SKK, Nektar, Centrexion, and Scilex. R. Nalamasu: Nothing to disclose.

REFERENCES

1. Institute of Medicine (US) Committee on Advancing Pain Research, Care, and Education. Relieving Pain in America: A Blueprint for Transforming Prevention, Care, Education, and Research. Washington (DC): National Academies Press; 2011. Available at: https://www.ncbi.nlm.nih.gov/books/NBK92525/.
2. The Forum at the Harvard T.H. Chan School of Public Health, The Huffington Post. "The chronic pain epidemic." The Forum at Harvard T. H. Chan School of Public Health, 15 Nov. 2017. Available at: theforum.sph.harvard.edu/events/the-chronic-pain-epidemic/. Accessed October 1, 2019.
3. Dahlhamer J, Lucas J, Zelaya C, et al. Prevalence of Chronic Pain and High-Impact Chronic Pain Among Adults — United States, 2016. MMWR Morb Mortal Wkly Rep 2018;67:1001–6.
4. Volkow N. Deep dive: the opioid tsunami: aspen ideas. Aspen Ideas Festival; 2017. Available at: www.aspenideas.org/sessions/deep-dive-the-opioid-tsunami?gclid=EAIaIQobChMI85ibsPH95AIVDdNkCh3jhAwyEAAYASAAEgKf_PD_BwE.
5. Available at: https://safety.nsc.org/prescription-nation-facing-americas-opioid-epidemic. Accessed October 03, 2019.
6. CDC, Center for Disease Control. Synthetic opioid overdose data. Centers for Disease Control and Prevention, Centers for Disease Control and Prevention; 2019. Available at: www.cdc.gov/drugoverdose/data/fentanyl.html.
7. Litman RS, Pagán OH, Cicero TJ. Abuse-deterrent opioid formulations. Anesthesiology 2018;128(5):1015–26.
8. Chung MK, Campbell JN. Use of capsaicin to treat pain: mechanistic and therapeutic considerations. Pharmaceuticals (Basel) 2016;9:66.
9. Derry S, Sven-Rice A, Cole P, et al. Topical capsaicin (High Concentration) for chronic neuropathic pain in adults. Cochrane Database Syst Rev 2013;(2):CD007393.
10. Derry S, Moore RA. Topical capsaicin (low concentration) for chronic neuropathic pain in adults. Prescriber 2012;23(19):24.
11. Stevens RM, Ervin J, Nezzer J, et al. Randomized, double-blind, placebo-controlled trial of intraarticulartrans- capsaicin for pain associated with osteoarthritis of the knee. Arthritis Rheumatol 2019;71(9):1524–33.
12. Centrexiontherapeutics, centrexion therapeutics."CNTX-4975". Centrexion; 2018. Available at: centrexion.com/science/pipeline/cntx-4975/.
13. Ramos M, Tatjana A, Atkinson TJ. Inside the potential of nerve growth factor antagonists. Pract Pain Management 2019;19(4):55–9.
14. Shelton DL, Zeller J, Ho WH, et al. Nerve growth factor mediates hyperalgesia and cachexia in auto-immune arthritis. Pain 2005;116(1):8–16.
15. Schnitzer TJ, Marks JA. A systematic review of the efficacy and general safety of antibodies to NGF in the treatment of OA of the hip or knee. Osteoarthritis Cartilage 2015;23. https://doi.org/10.1016/j.joca.2014.10.003.

16. Schnitzer TJ, Easton R, Pang S, et al. Effect of Tanezumab on joint pain, physical function, and patient global assessment of osteoarthritis among patients with osteoarthritis of the hip or knee. JAMA 2019;322(1):37.

17. Gimbel JS, Kivitz AJ, Bramson C, et al. Long-term safety and effectiveness of tanezumab as treatment for chronic low back pain. Pain 2014;155(9):1793–801.

18. Dakin P, DiMartino SJ, Gao H, et al. The efficacy, tolerability, and joint safety of fasinumab in osteoarthritis pain: a phase IIb/III double-blind, placebo-controlled, randomized clinical trial. ArthritisRheumatol 2019;71(11):1824–34.

19. Minett MS, Pereira V, Sikandar S, et al. Endogenous opioids contribute to insensitivity to pain in humans and mice lacking sodium channel Nav1.7. Nat Commun 2015;6(1):8967.

20. Offord C. Targeting sodium channels for pain relief. The Scientist Magazine® 2018. Available at: www.the-scientist.com/features/targeting-sodium-channels-for-pain-relief-30147.

21. Focken T, Liu S, Chahal N, et al. Discovery of aryl sulfonamides as isoform-selective inhibitors of Na-$_V$1.7 with efficacy in rodent pain models. ACS Med ChemLett 2016;7:277–82.

22. Shcherbatko A, Rossi A, Foletti D, et al. Engineering highly potent and selective microproteins against Nav1.7 sodium channel for treatment of pain. J Biol Chem 2016;291(27):13974–86.

23. Faber CG, Lauria G, Merkies IS, et al. Gain-of-function Nav1.8 mutations in painful neuropathy. ProcNatlAcadSci U S A 2012;109(47):19444–9.

24. Leipold E, Liebmann L, Korenke GC, et al. A de novo gain-of-function mutation in SCN11A causes loss of pain perception. Nat Genet 2013;45(11):1399–404.

25. Maher DP, Chen L, Mao J. Intravenous ketamine infusions for neuropathic pain management: a promising therapy inneed of optimization. Anesth Analg 2017;124(2):661–74.

26. Sigtermans MJ, van Hilten JJ, Bauer MCR, et al. Ketamine produces effective and long-term pain relief in patients with complex regional pain syndrome type 1. Pain 2009;145(3):304–11.

27. Kiefer R-T, Rohr P, Ploppa A, et al. Efficacy of ketamine in anesthetic dosage for the treatment of refractory complex regional pain syndrome: an open-label Phase II study. Pain Med 2008;9(8):1173–201.

28. Eichenberger U, Neff F, Sveticic G, et al. Chronic phantom limb pain: the effects of calcitonin, ketamine, and their combination on pain and sensory thresholds. AnesthAnalg 2008;106(4):1265–73.

29. Lynch ME, Clark AJ, Sawynok J, et al. Topical 2% amitriptyline and 1% ketamine in neuropathic pain syndromes: a randomized, double-blind, placebo-controlled trial. Anesthesiology 2005;103(1):140–6.

30. Rabi J, Minori J, Abad H, et al. Topical ketamine 10% for neuropathic pain in spinal cord injury patients: an open-label trial. Int J Pharm Compd 2016;20(6):517–20.

31. Mahoney JM, Vardaxis V, Moore JL, et al. Topical ketamine cream in the treatment of painful diabetic neuropathy: a randomized, placebo-controlled, double-blind initial study. J Am Podiatr Med Assoc 2012;102(3):178–83.

32. Aptinyx Inc., Aptinyx Inc. "Aptinyx to present preclinical data on three clinical-stage NMDA Receptor Modulators at the 49th Annual Meeting of the Society for Neuroscience." Aptinyx, 15 Oct. 2019, Available at: ir.aptinyx.com/news-releases/news-release-details/aptinyx-present-preclinical-data-three-clinical-stage-nmda.

33. Steiner D, Munera C, Hale M, et al. Efficacy and safety of Buprenorphine Trans-dermal System (BTDS) for chronic moderate to severe low back pain: a random-ized, double-blind study. J Pain 2011;12(11):1163–73.
34. Butrans [Package Insert]. Stamford (CT): Purdue Pharma L.P; 2014.
35. BioDelivery Sciences International, Inc. BELBUCA® (Buprenorphine) buccal film: rethink relief. Belbuca®; 2019. Available at:www.belbuca.com/.
36. Ge X, Henningfield JE, Siddhanti S, et al. Human abuse potential of oral NKTR-181 in recreational opioid users: a randomized, double-blind, crossover study. Pain Med 2019. https://doi.org/10.1093/pm/pnz232.
37. Tepper SJ. History and review of Anti-Calcitonin Gene-Related Peptide (CGRP) therapies: from translational research to treatment. Headache 2018;58:238–75.
38. Do TP, Guo S, Ashina M. Therapeutic novelties in migraine: new drugs, new hope? J Headache Pain 2019;20(1):37.
39. Croop R, Goadsby PJ, Stock DA, et al. Efficacy, safety, and tolerability of rimege-pant orally disintegrating tablet for the acute treatment of migraine: a rando-mised, phase 3, double-blind, placebo-controlled trial. Lancet 2019; 394(10200):737–45.
40. Trugman JM, et al. Efficacy, safety, and tolerability of ubrogepant for the acute treatment of migraine: results from a single-attack phase 3 study, ACHIEVE II (S38.008). Neurology 2019;92(15 supplement):38.008. Available at: n.neurology.org/content/92/15_Supplement/S38.008.
41. Dodick DW, et al. A.07 efficacy, safety, and tolerability of ubrogepant for the acute treatment of migraine: a single-attack phase 3 study, ACHIEVE I. Can J Neurol Sci 2019;46:s1.
42. Kohnen R, Krüger HP, Dulin J. The human-experimental investigation of sedative effects from drugs in combination with alcohol. Psycho 1995;21(12):768–75.
43. Dulin J, Kovacs L, Ramm S, et al. Evaluation of sedative effects of single and repeat doses of 50 mg and 150 mg TolperisoneHydohloride. Results of a pro-spective, randomized, doubleblind, placebo-controlled trial. Pharmakopsychiatr 1998;31:137–42.
44. Tekes K. Basic aspects of the pharmacodynamics of tolperisone, a widely appli-cable centrally acting muscle relaxant. Open Med Chem J 2014;8(1):17–22.
45. Kohne-Volland R. The clinical trial of Mydocalm (Tolperisone hydrochloride). Qual Clin Pract 2002;1:29–39.
46. Melka A, Tekle-Haimanot R, Lambien F, et al. Symptomatic treatment of neurola-thyrism with tolperisone (Mydocalm): a randomized double blind and placebo controlled drug trial. Ethiop Med J 1997;35(2):77–91.
47. Pratzel HG, Alken RG, Ramm S. Efficacy and tolerance of repeated oral doses of tolperisone hydrochloride in the treatment of painful reflex muscle spasm: results of a prospective placebo-controlled double-blind trial. Pain 1996;67(2):417–25.
48. Kameyama T, Nabeshima T, Sugimoto A, et al. Antinociceptiveaction of Tizani-dine in mice and rats. NaunynSchmiedebergs Arch Pharmacol 1985;330(2):93–6.
49. Sakitama K. The effects of centrally acting muscle relaxants on the intrathecal noradrenaline-induced facilitation of the flexor reflex mediated by group II afferent fibers in rats. Jpn J Pharmacol 1993;63(3):369–76.
50. Sakaue A, Honda M, Tanabe M, et al. Antinociceptive effects of sodium channel-blocking agents on acute pain in mice. J Pharmacol Sci 2004;95(2):181–8.
51. Chiba K, Matsuyama Y, Seo T, et al. Condoliase for the treatment of lumbar disc herniation. Spine (Phila Pa 1976) 2018;43(15):E869–76. Available at: https://www. ncbi.nlm.nih.gov/pubmed/29257028. Accessed May 7, 2019.

52. Kaken Pharmaceutical Co, Ltd. Seikagaku and Kaken announce the launch of HERNICORE®1.25 units for intradiscal injection in Japan, indicated for treatment of lumbar disc herniation. Kaken Pharmaceutical Co.,Ltd.; 2018. Available at: www.kaken.co.jp/english/en_release/seikagaku-and-kaken-announce-the-launch-of-hernicore1-25-units-for-intradiscal-injection-in-japanindicated-for-treatment-of-lumbar-disc-herniation.html.

Nonsteroidal Antiinflammatory Drugs for Acute and Chronic Pain

Timothy J. Atkinson, PharmD, BCPS, CPE[a],*,
Jeffrey Fudin, BS, PharmD, FCCP, FFSMB[b,c,d]

KEYWORDS

- NSAIDs • Chronic pain • Stiffness • Inflammation • Adjuvant analgesics
- Nonopioid

KEY POINTS

- Nonsteroidal antiinflammatory drugs (NSAIDs) represent a key strategy in nonopioid pharmacologic management of nociceptive pain.
- Expected benefits of NSAIDs include reducing stiffness and inflammation, and improving mobility.
- NSAID use is widespread and should be monitored to avoid or mitigate risks of gastrointestinal bleeding, renal dysfunction, or cardiovascular events.
- Topical NSAIDs are underused and often preferred to oral NSAIDs because of similar efficacy over a localized area with minimal risk of systemic toxicity.

INTRODUCTION

An estimated 23% of US adults (54 million) were diagnosed with some form of arthritis (includes osteoarthritis [OA], gout, lupus, and rheumatoid arthritis) between 2013 and 2015, and nearly 10% (24 million) reported arthritis-attributable activity limitations. Arthritis is also the leading cause of work disability in the United States, with 6.4% (15 million) reporting severe joint pain caused by arthritis. By 2040, the number of US adults diagnosed with arthritis is projected to increase by 44% (78 million) as a result of an aging population.[1] It is no surprise that nonsteroidal antiinflammatory drugs (NSAIDs) have dominated the treatment of arthritis for the last century, with nearly 50% of NSAID prescriptions being written for OA.[2] Including over-the-counter (OTC) NSAID use, an estimated 12.8% of the US population

[a] Pain Management, PGY2 Pain Management & Palliative Care Pharmacy Residency, VA Tennessee Valley Healthcare System, 3400 Lebanon Pike, Murfreesboro, TN 37129, USA; [b] Pain Management, PGY2 Pain Management & Palliative Care Pharmacy Residency, Albany Stratton VA Medical Center, 113 Holland Avenue, Albany, NY 12208, USA; [c] Albany College of Pharmacy and Health Sciences, Albany, NY, USA; [d] Remitigate LLC, Delmar, NY, USA
* Corresponding author.
E-mail address: Timothy.atkinson@va.gov

Phys Med Rehabil Clin N Am 31 (2020) 219–231
https://doi.org/10.1016/j.pmr.2020.01.002
1047-9651/20/Published by Elsevier Inc.

uses NSAIDs regularly, which is double the number of people on chronic opioid therapy.[3]

The effectiveness of NSAIDs was established long ago. However, even in modern times, when measuring the efficacy of NSAIDs in knee osteoarthritis, NSAIDs are 3 times more effective at controlling stiffness and inflammation, and improving mobility, compared with acetaminophen despite the latter being recommended more often because of perceived safety.[4] Regardless, for the past several decades, studies evaluating NSAIDs have focused almost exclusively on their adverse effects and attempts to mitigate them. Clinicians are therefore constantly barraged with the risk of adverse effects, resulting in avoidance or inability to determine the place of NSAIDs in therapy. Without reviewing the history of NSAIDs, it can be difficult to reconcile recent evidence with efficacy to balance their risks and benefits in modern treatment paradigms.

HISTORY

Salicylic acid was first derived from willow bark in the form of salicin by Johann Buchner in 1828, but willow bark had been used medicinally for centuries because of its antipyretic and antiinflammatory properties. An Italian chemist named Raffaele Piria made the next scientific breakthrough around 1838 when he produced a more active and pure form of salicylic acid, paving the way for broader use in medicine. Salicylic acid was then used effectively to treat rheumatoid arthritis, rheumatic fever, gout, and other inflammatory and arthritic conditions over the next few decades. The first form of acetylsalicylic acid (ASA) was created by buffering it with sodium and acetyl chloride in 1853 by Francis Gerhardt, the French chemist. However, his research effort was abandoned because he failed to recognize the potential benefits, including improved gastrointestinal (GI) tolerance. Although salicylic acid use was common during this era, Felix Hoffman created a more stable form of acetylsalicylic acid and it was marketed in 1899 by Bayer under the tradename Aspirin. Aspirin quickly became the most widely used painkiller worldwide, commonly used for arthritis, headaches, and back pain.[5] Rheumatology treatment guidelines from 1939 reinforce the profound impact the first antiinflammatories had on the treatment and management of rheumatic and arthritic conditions. The guidelines state, "…because of its antipyretic action in rheumatic fever, because of its analgesic property, because of its relative harmlessness and ready accessibility, it has won a place in the armoury of the attack on rheumatism that has scarcely been challenged."[6] By then, the efficacy of NSAIDs was well established, and NSAIDs profoundly changed practice at a time when opioids were widely available and largely unregulated. Most people alive now do not remember the doses of salicylic acid required to treat serious inflammatory and rheumatic conditions, but before the modern age of NSAIDs it was common to use up to 5.2 g (16 tablets) daily for rheumatoid arthritis, and even higher for rheumatic fever, with 12 g daily (37 tablets). Doses of salicylic acid were often escalated until patients complained of tinnitus (ringing in the ears) and were then instructed to decrease by 1 tablet each day until it resolved.[7] GI intolerance was common but there were few alternative treatment options and therefore salicylic acid remained the preferred treatment option. However, ingestion of large amounts of salicylic acid had consequences, and it was common for patients to develop a serious acid/base imbalance called salicylism (a toxic and serious adverse effect caused by high serum levels of salicylate with symptoms of tinnitus, vomiting, and nausea), resulting in respiratory alkalosis, which is characterized by cramps and/or weakness. In 1 trial of patients being treated for rheumatic fever, the incidence of salicyism was 80% of those enrolled receiving ASA.[7]

With the approval of indomethacin in 1965, a new era of NSAID research and therapy commenced. Although indomethacin is now known to cause a higher risk of GI ulcers and bleeding because of its overwhelming cyclooxygenase (COX) 1 selectivity, at the time of its approval, it was a major step forward in pharmacotherapy because of reduced overall pill burden, acid load, and general GI tolerability.[5] The mechanism of action for NSAIDs was first successfully described and confirmed by a British pharmacologist, Sir John Vane, who in 1982 won a Nobel Prize for his work. An increased understanding of the mechanism of action for NSAIDs ushered in a time of innovation and rapid development, a sort of NSAID renaissance, from 1976 to 1992 with more than 15 new NSAIDs developed and marketed. There are currently more than 25 NSAIDs available from 6 distinct pharmacologic classes, each with its own unique receptor selectivity, pharmacokinetics, and adverse effects.[8]

NONSTEROIDAL ANTIINFLAMMATORY DRUG CHEMICAL CLASSES
Pharmacology

NSAIDs are valuable therapeutic agents for their ability to reduce pain, fever, and inflammation through inhibition of prostaglandin synthesis at COX enzymes (**Fig. 1**).[9] There are 2 forms of COX enzymes: COX-1 is constitutively expressed in all cells, whereas COX-2 expression is generally induced at the site of tissue injury, but they each have distinct roles physiologically. COX-1 enzymes are responsible for regulating GI cytoprotection, platelet function, and renal function, and produce thromboxane (TXA2) and prostacyclin (PGI2) in equal amounts to maintain a balance.[10,11] Both NSAIDs and ASA share the same catalytic site, and binding results in increasing bleeding risk by suppressing platelet function. Although they share the same binding site, there are important differences in their binding kinetics, with clinical and therapeutic implications. NSAIDs bind competitively, resulting in limited bleeding risk corresponding with exposure and half-life, whereas ASA binds covalently (irreversibly) to serine 529 near the catalytic site but blocks it permanently, resulting in profoundly

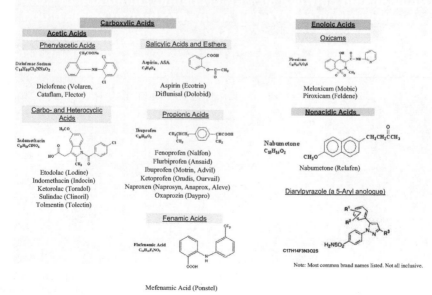

Fig. 1. Chemical classes of NSAIDs in the United States. (*Courtesy* J. Fudin, BS, PharmD, DAAPM, FCCP, Albany, NY.)

increased bleeding risk even at lower doses because platelets are inhibited for their entire life cycle (7–10 days). This property of ASA has transformed its modern use into a cardioprotective agent (antiplatelet) that has the ability to fully inhibit platelet function at dosages as low as 40 mg/d with chronic use.[10] COX-2 enzymes are responsible for inflammation, pain, and fever, making them preferred targets in pain management. COX-2 is induced by cytokine release from injury and/or inflammation; however, they are also constitutively expressed in the brain, kidneys, and blood vessels, sites that are highly susceptible to thrombotic events.[12–16] COX selectivity and binding characteristics are strongly associated with their adverse event profile.

Pharmacokinetics

NSAIDs have unique pharmacokinetics that are critical to understanding their potential adverse effects and how to mitigate them. As a class, NSAIDs are all greater than 90% protein bound, and with only the free fraction of circulating drug able to exert its pharmacologic effect. Adverse effects such as GI bleeds, renal impairment, and thrombotic effects can be dramatically increased when the amount bound to proteins is disrupted via drug interactions or severe hepatic function and declining ability to produce plasma proteins. NSAIDs are known to cause local toxicity in the GI tract regardless of COX selectivity because they are all weak acids and can be corrosive and erode at protective barriers. COX-1 inhibitors compound this problem with antagonizing protective prostaglandins increasing risk of GI bleeds. NSAIDs are often formulated to minimize this risk with enteric coating, buffered formulations, antacids, or addition of misoprostol, but this is often insufficient and some patients require gastric protection through prophylactic treatment, generally with proton pump inhibitors (PPIs), which have shown benefit by protecting against both peptic and duodenal ulcers.[17] **Fig. 2** shows that the COX selectivity of NSAIDs is not absolute and each

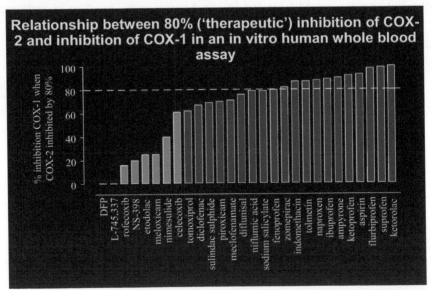

Fig. 2. COX selectivity of NSAIDs. DFP; (3-(2-propyloxy)-4-(4-methylsulphonylphenyl)-5,5-dimethylfuranone. (*From* Warner TD, Giuliano F, Vojnovic I, et al. Nonsteroid drug selectivities for cyclo-oxygenase-1 rather than cyclo-oxygenase-2 are associated with human gastrointestinal toxicity: A full *in vitro* analysis. PNAS. 1999; 96(13):7563-7568; with permission.)

NSAID has some level of inhibition of both COX-1 and COX-2, which is a critical concept because they lose selectivity at high doses, resulting in maximum inhibition of both COX isoenzymes.[18] Another common characteristic of NSAIDs is their metabolism as a class through the cytochrome P (CYP) 2C9 enzyme system. 2C9 does not have the same risk of drug interactions as other more common CYP 450 enzymes (3A4 or 2D6), but 2C9 is highly polymorphic and susceptible to both drug interactions and phenotype expression affecting efficacy.[19,20]

INTERVENTIONAL PROCEDURES AND NONSTEROIDAL ANTIINFLAMMATORY DRUG DISCONTINUATION

To minimize bleeding risk before an interventional procedure or surgery, patients are often required to discontinue NSAID therapy. These instructions to patients often follow preset protocols requiring discontinuing NSAID therapy 7 to 10 days before the intervention. This recommendation is traceable to projected platelet inhibition after ASA but is excessively conservative and may result in needless suffering for those patients that rely on NSAID use for decreased stiffness, inflammation, and improved mobility.[21] All NSAIDs, other than acetylsalicylic acid, inhibit platelet function and by extension increase bleeding risk only for the duration of their pharmacologic effects.

Pharmacokinetics can assist with prediction of bleeding risk using the half-life of the medication. It takes 5 half-lives for the body to completely excrete the drug from the body and, when it is absent, it can no longer exert a pharmacologic effect. For example, ibuprofen has a half-life of 2 hours, indicating that after 2 hours 50% of the drug has been eliminated from circulation and is no longer active. Therefore, a more practical approach would be discontinuing each agent according to its bleeding risk and/or after 5 half-lives, which in the case of ibuprofen means that, within 24 hours of the last dose, any bleeding risk disappeared along with the drug when it was completely eliminated from the body. When the exact bleeding risk is unknown, the American Society of Regional Anesthesia is in agreement with this approach, recommending discontinuing NSAID therapy 5 half-lives before the scheduled procedure.[22] More recently, comprehensive consensus guidelines were developed collaboratively by the American Society of Regional Anesthesia and Pain Medicine, the European Society of Regional Anesthesia and Pain Therapy, the American Academy of Pain Medicine, the International Neuromodulation Society, the North American Neuromodulation Society, and the World Institute of Pain that systematically outline practical considerations for continuing or discontinuing various medications, and the timing of therapy restoration for individual drugs and pharmacologic drug classes that warrant consideration for planned intraspinal procedures. These drugs include non-ASA NSAIDs, ASA, phosphodiesterase inhibitors, glycoprotein IIb/IIIa inhibitors, antidepressants and serotonin reuptake inhibitors, P2Y12 inhibitors (ticlopidine, clopidogrel, prasugrel, ticagrelor, cangrelor), coumarol-based anticoagulants, heparin and low-molecular-weight heparin, thrombolytic agents, and novel oral anticoagulants.[23] This approach allows clinicians to tailor therapy to the individual patient without compromising on safety concerns.

FOOD AND DRUG ADMINISTRATION WARNINGS

There have been 2 major updates to US Food and Drug Administration (FDA)–approved labeling in the form of FDA warnings. In 2005, the FDA released a box warning for all NSAIDs, stating that (1) NSAIDs are associated with an increased risk of adverse cardiovascular thrombotic events, including myocardial infarction and stroke; and (2) NSAIDs may increase risk of GI irritation, inflammation, ulceration, bleeding, and perforation. These events may occur at any time during therapy and without warning. In July 2015, the FDA strengthened warnings for cardiovascular events with NSAIDs as a class effect after a meta-analysis of high-dose NSAID use showed significant cardiovascular risk even in NSAIDs more selective for COX-1.[24]

GASTROINTESTINAL ADVERSE EFFECTS

In 1999, the prevalence of annual deaths attributable to NSAID-related GI bleeds was around 16,500, and, although still widely referenced today, national tracking of causes of death have provided revised estimates.[25] In 2009, the number of deaths attributed to GI bleeds was 7215, of which one-third can be attributed to NSAID use.[26] Providers should be aware that a history of ulcers, *Helicobacter pylori* infection, older age, and higher doses of NSAIDs can be risk factors for GI injury. Roughly 30% of GI bleeds are attributable to ASA alone.[27] To avoid increased bleeding risk, patients should be counseled to avoid OTC NSAIDs/aspirin coadministration with prescription NSAIDs.[9]

COX-1 inhibition directly affects platelet aggregation, and the degree of COX-1 inhibition predicts bleeding risk.[16,28] Because NSAIDs bind reversibly to COX-1, they inhibit platelet function only for the duration of binding and must be taken consistently to increase risk of bleeding. NSAIDs highly selective for COX-1 (>50 times more COX-1 selective) consistently result in more GI ulcers and bleeding. Examples include ketorolac, piroxicam, sulindac, and indomethacin (**Fig. 3**).[9,26,29] Minimizing risk requires familiarity with these properties and effective use of gastroprotective therapy to ensure effectiveness while minimizing risk to patients. Strategies to provide gastroprotection include choosing a more COX-2–selective NSAID and/or coadministration of PPIs or misoprostol, both of which have significant evidence to reduce both gastric and duodenal ulcers.[17]

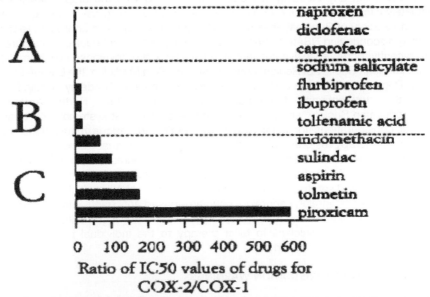

Fig. 3. COX-1 selectivity. Group A = equipotent inhibitors of COX-1/COX-2; group B = 10 to 50 times more potent COX-1 inhibition; group C = greater than 50 times COX-1 inhibition. IC50, half maximal inhibitory concentration. (*Modified from* Mitchell JA, Larkin S, Williams TJ. Cyclooxygenase-2: regulation and relevance in inflammation. *Biochem Pharmacol.* 1995; 50(10):1535-1542; with permission.)

CARDIOVASCULAR EVENTS

Antiinflammatories are used almost exclusively for their COX-2 properties with intent to target the deleterious effects of inflammation, pain, and fever. Because these are all mediated by COX-2, it would require much higher doses of COX-1–selective NSAIDs to achieve a level of COX-2 inhibition sufficient to provide benefit, further increasing bleeding risk. The research effort into COX-2–selective NSAIDs was the natural extension of the intent to directly target specific symptoms. In theory, NSAIDs with greater COX-2 selectivity would have increased analgesic benefits while decreasing bleeding risk. The first 2 highly selective COX-2 inhibitors, often referred to as coxibs, were highly successful and quickly dominated the market for NSAIDs. Early studies raised concerns about potentially increased cardiovascular risk, resulting in the FDA requiring specific studies to determine the cardiovascular risk of these agents. Rofecoxib (Vioxx) and valdecoxib (Bextra) were both voluntarily removed from the market as a result of those studies seeming to confirm thromboembolic risk.[30,31]

The current theory on the mechanism for increased thromboembolic risk with COX-2–selective NSAIDs is disruption of the prostacyclin and thromboxane balance by disproportionately inhibiting prostacyclin. There has also been significant concern that refusal to allow patients access to low-dose ASA for its cardioprotective benefits, even when they had previous cardiac events, may have skewed the results. In 2017, a meta-analysis evaluating NSAID-related cardiovascular risk was published reviewing the impact of those early coxib studies. The investigators removed the rofecoxib data from those trials and evaluated whether the coxibs without rofecoxib significantly increased risk of cardiovascular events. When rofecoxib's data were removed from the coxib group, the cardiovascular risk of coxibs versus traditional NSAIDs was no longer statistically significant, and this seems to indicate that the rofecoxib studies may have significantly skewed the data.[32] This finding raises questions about whether the removal of these agents was premature. There are several coxibs available in Europe that are not available in the United States, including parecoxib, an intravenous (IV) prodrug of valdecoxib.

Although the debate over whether coxibs increase cardiovascular events more than traditional NSAIDs has gained new life, there is no question that NSAIDs as a class do increase risk of cardiovascular events, particularly among patients with a history of cardiac events. Several meta-analyses reinforce the cardiovascular risk of NSAIDs and require providers to be thoughtful about their use.[33,34] Some COX-2 selectivity is ideal; however, the authors advise counseling patients on the realistic benefits of NSAID therapy while using the lowest effective dose. Oral NSAIDs should be avoided in patients with a history or serious risk of thromboembolic events (stroke or myocardial infarction).

ADVERSE EFFECTS

The effects of widespread inappropriate use of NSAIDs are underestimated and potentially inflate the risk of taking NSAIDs as recommended. Large population-based surveys have provided some alarming results on NSAID use. Forty percent of patients prescribed NSAIDs also report taking an OTC NSAID on a regular basis.[35] Twenty-nine percent believe that OTC NSAIDs are safer than prescription NSAIDs, and 16% report taking NSAIDs and ASA together, further increasing bleeding risk.[26,35] Patient education on safe use of NSAIDs is encouraged and necessary to mitigate unintentional adverse effects.

For the past 20 years, NSAID research and new drug approvals have focused heavily on mitigating their adverse effects. The level of COX inhibition and the balance between prostacyclin and thromboxane remains a popular theory regarding prediction of adverse effects.[10,36] Decades of research have led to a few conclusions regarding NSAID dosing and temporal relationship with the potential adverse effects. All NSAIDs tend to lose COX selectivity at higher doses. The risk of GI events nearly doubles with high-dose NSAID therapy compared with low/moderate doses of NSAIDs. Cardiovascular risk is only marginally affected by NSAID dose. Risk of renal impairment increases by roughly 50% at higher doses compared with low/moderate doses.[37–39] Few studies have evaluated the impact of chronic NSAID use, and the duration of NSAID therapy can be as relevant as the dose in predicting adverse effects. The highest risk of GI adverse events seems to be in the first 14 days of therapy. Cardiovascular risk is not significantly affected by duration of therapy. Risk of renal failure seems to increase over time, perhaps indicating a type of cumulative effect over time.[39–41]

TOPICAL NONSTEROIDAL ANTIINFLAMMATORY DRUGS

The increased attention on the consequences of oral NSAID use has led to increasing recommendations to use topical NSAIDs; however, these agents have the same class effect warnings for GI bleeds, renal impairment, and cardiovascular risk as other NSAIDs, leading to confusion and poor use. However, similar to oral formulations, topical NSAIDs have significant evidence to improve function and decrease stiffness for those with osteoarthritis, with an effect size 3 times larger than acetaminophen, and they are superior to opioids in restoring and promoting mobility.[4] Topical NSAIDs administered over a localized area can achieve tissue concentrations several times higher than oral administration.[42] Recent guidelines for hand and knee osteoarthritis have begun to favor topical NSAID use rather than oral because of similar efficacy with far less risk of systemic adverse effects.[43–45]

In Europe, there are several topical NSAIDs that have been available for use for decades, but in the United States the only topical NSAID available other than salicylate derivatives is diclofenac by prescription only, in several formulations at the time of publication. Although compounding pharmacies may create topical analgesic creams using ketoprofen, piroxicam, sulindac, or ibuprofen, these are not FDA approved for topical use. Topical NSAIDs can be effective because of their ability to inhibit COX enzymes locally and peripherally, without significant risk for systemic absorption. See the results of pharmacokinetic comparison of oral versus topical diclofenac serum concentrations in **Table 1**. The minimum systemic concentration of diclofenac required to decrease platelet aggregation by 40% is 400 ng/mL, which is difficult to achieve with a topical NSAID even at maximum recommended doses.[42] The maximum serum concentrations (Cmax) are also considerably less than known NSAID drug response indicators for effectiveness or IC50 (half maximal inhibitory concentrations) values for both COX-1 and COX-2, indicating that it is unlikely to achieve receptor activation.[46]

The FDA requires class effect warnings on topical NSAIDs, which continues to confuse and discourage providers from appropriate prescribing. A true understanding of the prevalence of adverse effects related to topical versus oral NSAID use would result in providers recognizing that topical NSAIDs can be particularly useful for localized pain complaints in patients who should not be using oral NSAIDs for safety reasons. Australia's Therapeutic Goods Administration performed a thorough safety review of diclofenac products in 2014. They queried the European Adverse Drug Reporting System, which is similar to the FDA Adverse Event Reporting System. There were 84 total reports of adverse events with topical diclofenac, but, when oral diclofenac was excluded, there remained only 3 total reports. One report was for GI bleed,

Table 1
Pharmacokinetic comparison of topical versus oral prescription diclofenac formulations

Diclofenac Prescription Dosage Forms						
Brand Name	Form	Strength	Dosage	Cmax (ng/mL)	Tmax (h)	AUC (ng/h/mL)
Diclofenac (Voltaren, Cataflam, generic)	Tablets	50 mg	TID	2270 ± 778	6.5	3890 ± 1710
Voltaren	Gel	1%	48 g/d[a]	53.8 ± 32	10	807 ± 478
Solaraze	Gel	3%	2g TID × 6 d	5 ± 5	4.5 ± 8	9 ± 19
Flector	Patch	1.3%	BID × 5 d	1.3–8.8	120	96
Pennsaid	Topical solution	1.5% w/w	QID × 7 d	19.4 ± 9.3	4 ± 6.5	745.2 ± 374.7

Abbreviations: AUC, area under the curve; BID, twice a day; Cmax, maximum serum concentration; QID, 4 times a day; TID, 3 times a day; Tmax, time required for a drug to achieve its peak plasma concentration.
[a] This is more than the maximum daily dose recommended.

and the other 2 were increased liver function tests, and, in their final report, they concluded, "Based on the available information the risk/benefit for topical diclofenac remains favorable. There is a paucity of evidence of serious systemic side effects with topical diclofenac."[47] The pharmacokinetic evidence combined with the postmarketing surveillance results makes it clear that topical NSAIDs simply do not have anywhere near the same level of risk of adverse events as oral NSAIDs.

NANO–NONSTEROIDAL ANTIINFLAMMATORY DRUGS

The most recent trend in FDA approvals for prescription NSAIDs has been micronized NSAIDs using nanotechnology. Micronized NSAIDs reduce particle size, increasing surface area for absorption, improving dissolution, and leading to quicker onset of analgesia at lower than traditional doses.[48] Submicrometer NSAIDs have much finer particles (approximately 10 times smaller than conventional formulations). Absorption of traditional NSAIDs is already high, leading many clinicians to question whether this will make any measurable clinical impact. To date, these submicrometer NSAIDs have shown the ability to achieve the same pharmacokinetic targets for efficacy (ie, Cmax), in addition to improving on predictors of adverse effects (area under the curve [AUC] and dose). For example, micronized diclofenac can achieve the same Cmax at 35 mg compared with 50 mg of the traditional formulation with decreased AUC.[48] Indomethacin similarly achieves the same Cmax at 40 mg compared with 50 mg of the traditional indomethacin.[49] Comparable efficacy has led to drug approval of several of these submicrometer NSAID formulations, but whether these pharmacokinetic targets will be accurate surrogate markers for reduced adverse effects remains to be confirmed with their required postmarketing studies.

Parenteral

In the United States, there are 2 IV NSAIDs available for pain at the time of publication. Ketorolac is the most well known and is widely used for short-term relief of severe acute pain in the emergency department, where it has shown similar effectiveness to IV opioids in several trials. The FDA-approved indication for ketorolac is unique among all NSAIDs because it is approved for the short-term (up to 5 days) management of moderate to severe acute pain at the opioid level.[50] This approval is significant for a few reasons: it reinforces that IV administration can provide profound relief even in a formulation known to be more than 50 times more COX-1 selective. However, its selectivity also results in a very high bleeding risk even among NSAIDs.[9] The 5-day limit to administration comes from a randomized clinical trial comparing ketorolac administered every 6 hours with opioid therapy and measured incidence of bleeding. Similar risk of bleeding was observed in both groups until day 5, whereas any longer duration resulted in profound increase in bleeding risk.[51] However, if an IV NSAID more selective for COX-2 were developed and the risk of bleeding could be minimized while preserving its profound effectiveness for targeting pain, then the health care system might be in a better position to address acute or perioperative pain. For completeness, ketorolac tomethamine nasal spray can also be included as an alternative to IV ketorolac in the outpatient setting.[52,53] The second IV NSAID formulation approved in the United States is ibuprofen (Caldolor), which is approved for mild to moderate pain, the management of moderate to severe pain as an adjunct to opioid analgesics, and the reduction of fever.[52] IV ibuprofen was studied in the perioperative setting, where it showed modest opioid-sparing potential without a significant increase in bleeding risk. Of note, IV meloxicam has completed and published phase III trials and, at the time of this publication, is being worked on by the FDA on drug labeling required for approval, and its progress will be watched with great interest.[54]

SUMMARY

NSAIDs represent the cornerstone of pain management for connective tissue disorders. They provide a significant advantage in the treatment and management of stiffness and inflammation, and improve mobility in otherwise crippling disease states. Their cardiovascular, renal, and GI risks are real but should be reviewed on an individual basis with an understanding of how comorbid conditions, dose, and length of therapy affect these risks. When chronic long-term treatment is required, NSAIDs provide significant advantages compared with the known toxicities of traditional steroids. Topical NSAIDs may be preferred to oral NSAIDs for localized inflammatory disorders with decreased risk of adverse effects because of limited systemic absorption. Clinicians must weigh the risks and benefits of NSAID use, whether chronic or intermittent, and consider the importance of addressing the underlying cause of pain to provide targeted pharmacotherapy and augment treatment.

DISCLOSURE

Both authors perform consulting activities with pharmaceutical manufacturers, among others, but none involved in manufacturing NSAIDs or competing products. Therefore, the authors have nothing to disclose.

REFERENCES

1. CDC. Arthritis-related statistics. 2018. Available at: https://www.cdc.gov/arthritis/data_statistics/arthritis-related-stats.htm. Accessed November 15, 2019.
2. Heyneman C, Lawless-Liday C, Wall G. Oral versus topical NSAIDs in rheumatic diseases a comparison. Drugs 2000;60(3):555–74.
3. Zhou Y, Boudreau DM, Freedman AN. Trends in the use of aspirin and nonsteroidal anti-inflammatory drugs in the general U.S. population. Pharmacoepidemiol Drug Saf 2014;23(1):43–50.

4. Zhang W, Moskowitz R, Abramson S, et al. OARSI recommendations for the management of hip and knee osteoarthritis Part III: changes in evidence following systematic cumulative update of research published through January 2009. Osteoarthritis Cartilage 2010;18:476–99.

5. Ugurlucan M, Caglar IM, Turhan N, et al. Aspirin: from a historical perspective. Recent Pat Cardiovasc Drug Discov 2012;7(1):71–6.

6. Tegner WS. The treatment of rheumatic diseases in the United States and the continent of Europe. Ann Rheum Dis 1939;1:249–303.

7. Farber H, Yiengst M, Shock N. Therapeutic Effect of therapeutic doses of aspirin on the acid-base balance of the blood in normal adults. Bethesda (MD): National Institute of Health; 1949.

8. Atkinson TJ, Fudin J, Jahn HL, et al. What's new in NSAID pharmacotherapy: oral agents to injectables. Pain Med 2013;14(S1):S11–7.

9. Conaghan PG. A turbulent decade for NSAIDs: update on current concepts of classification, epidemiology, comparative efficacy, and toxicity. Rheumatol Int 2012;32(6):1491–502.

10. Mitchell JA, Larkin S, Williams TJ. Cyclooxygenase-2: regulation and relevance in inflammation. Biochem Pharmacol 1995;50(10):1535–42.

11. Solomon GD. Nonopioid and adjuvant analgesics. In: Tollison CD, Satterthwaite JR, Tollison JW, editors. Practical pain management. Philadelphia: Lippincott Williams & Wilkins; 2002. p. 243–52.

12. Komhoff M, Grone H, Klein T, et al. Localization of cyclooxygenase-1 and -2 in adult and fetal human kidney: implication for renal function. Am J Physiol 1997; 272:F460–8.

13. Guan Y, Chang M, Cho W, et al. Cloning, expression, and regulation of rabbit cyclooxygenase-2 in renal medullary interstitial cells. Am J Physiol 1997;273: F18–26.

14. Yang T, Singh I, Pham H, et al. Regulation of cyclooxygenase expression in the kidney by dietary salt intake. Am J Physiol 1998;274:F481–9.

15. Harris RC, McKenna JA, Akai Y, et al. Cyclooxygenase-2 is associated with the macula densa of rat kidney and increases with salt restriction. J Clin Invest 1994;94:2504–10.

16. Brock TG, McNish RW, Peters-Golden M. Arachidonic acid is preferentially metabolized by cyclooxygenase-2 to prostacyclin and prostaglandin E2. J Biol Chem 1999;274(17):11660–6.

17. Rostom A, Dube C, Wells GA, et al. Prevention of NSAID-induced gastroduodenal ulcers. Cochrane Database Syst Rev 2002;(4):CD002296.

18. Warner T, Giuliano F, Vojnovic I, et al. Nonsteroidal drug selectivities for cyclo-oxygenase-1 rather than cyclo-oxygenase-2 are associated with human gastrointestinal toxicity: a full in vitro analysis. Proc Natl Acad Sci U S A 1999;96(13): 7563–8.

19. Cavallari L, Limdi N. Warfarin pharmacogenomics. Curr Opin Mol Ther 2009; 11(3):243–51.

20. Ma J, Lee K, Kuo G. Clinical application of pharmacogenomics. J Pharm Pract 2012;25(4):417–27.

21. Younan M, Atkinson TJ, Fudin J. A practical approach to discontinuing NSAID therapy prior to a procedure. Pract Pain Manag 2013;13(10):45–51.

22. Horlocker TT, Wedel DJ, Rowlingson JC, et al. Regional anesthesia in the patient receiving antithrombotic or thrombolytic therapy: American Society of Regional Anesthesia and Pain Medicine evidence-/based guidelines (3rd Edition). Reg Anesth Pain Med 2009;35(1):64–101.

23. Narouze S, Benzon HT, Provenzano D, et al. Interventional spine and pain procedures in patients on antiplatelet and anticoagulant medications: guidelines from the American Society of regional anesthesia and Pain medicine, the European Society of regional anaesthesia and pain therapy, the American Academy of pain medicine, the International neuromodulation Society, the North American neuromodulation Society, and the world Institute of pain. Reg Anesth Pain Med 2018;43(3):225–62.

24. FDA. FDA Drug Safety Communication: FDA strengthens warning that non-aspirin nonsteroidal anti-inflammatory drugs (NSAIDs) can cause heart attacks or strokes. 2015. Available at: https://www.fda.gov/drugs/drug-safety-and-availability/fda-drug-safety-communication-fda-strengthens-warning-non-aspirin-nonsteroidal-anti-inflammatory. Accessed November 9, 2019.

25. Singh G, Triadafilopoulos G. Epidemiology of NSAID induced gastrointestinal complications. J Rheumatol 1999;26(Suppl 56):18–24.

26. Peery AF, Dellon ES, Lund J, et al. Burden of gastrointestinal disease in the United States: 2012 update. Gastroenterology 2012;143(5):1179–87.

27. Sorensen HT, Mellemkjaer L, Blot WJ, et al. Risk of upper gastrointestinal bleeding associated with use of low-dose aspirin. Am J Gastroenterol 2000; 95(9):2218–24.

28. Schafer AI. Effects of nonsteroidal antiinflammatory drugs on platelet function and systemic hemostasis. J Clin Pharmacol 1995;35:209–19.

29. Rainsford KD. An analysis of the gastrointestinal side effects of nonsteroidal anti-inflammatory drugs, with particular reference to comparative studies in man and laboratory species. Rheumatol Int 1983;2:1–10.

30. Bombardier C, Laine L, Reicin A, et al. Comparison of upper gastrointestinal toxicity of rofecoxib and naproxen in patients with rheumatoid arthritis. N Engl J Med 2000;343:1520–8.

31. Nussmeier N, Whelton A, Brown M, et al. Safety and efficacy of the cyclooxygenase-2 inhibitors parecoxib and valdecoxib after noncardiac surgery. Anesthesiology 2006;104(3):518–26.

32. Gunter BR, Butler KA, Wallace RL, et al. NSAID-induced CV adverse events. J Clin Pharm Ther 2017;42:27–38.

33. Bhala N, Emberson J, Merhi A, et al. Vascular and upper gastrointestinal effects of nonsteroidal anti-inflammatory drugs: meta-analysis of individual participant data from randomized trials. Lancet 2013;382(9894):769–79.

34. Trelle S, Reichenbach S, Wandel S, et al. Cardiovascular safety of non-steroidal anti-inflammatory drugs: network meta-analysis. BMJ 2011;342:c7086.

35. Wilcox CM, Cryer B, Triadafilopoulos G. Patterns of use and public perception of over-the-counter pain relievers: focus on nonsteroidal antiinflammatory drugs. J Rheumatol 2005;32(11):2218–24.

36. Cheng Y, Austin S, Rocca B, et al. Role of prostacyclin in the cardiovascular response to thromboxane A2. Science 2002;296:539–41.

37. Garcia Rodriguez LA, Hernandez-Diaz S. Relative risk of upper gastrointestinal complications among users of acetaminophen and nonsteroidal anti-inflammatory drugs. Epidemiology 2001;12(5):570–6.

38. Garcia Rodriguez L, Taconelli S, Patrignani P, et al. Role of dose potency in the prediction of risk of myocardial infarction associated with non-steroidal anti-inflammatory drugs in the general population. J Am Coll Cardiol 2008;52(120): 1628–36.

39. Huerta C, Castellsague J, Varas-Lorenzo C, et al. Nonsteroidal anti-inflammatory drugs and risk of ARF in the general population. Am J Kidney Dis 2005;45(3):531–9.
40. Helin-Salmivaara A, Saarelaninen S, Gronroos J, et al. Risk of upper gastrointestinal events with the use of various NSAIDs. Scand J Gastroenterol 2007;42(8):923–32.
41. Helin-Salmivaara A, Virtanen A, Vesalainen R, et al. NSAID use and the risk of hospitalization for first myocardial infarction in the general population: a nationwide case–control study from Finland. Eur Heart J 2006;27(14):1657–63.
42. Petersen B, Rovati S. Diclofenac epolamine (Flector®) patch evidence for topical activity. Clin Drug Invest 2009;29(1):1–9.
43. Hochberg M, Altman R, April K, et al. American College of Rheumatology 2012 recommendations for the use of nonpharmacologic and pharmacologic therapies in osteoarthritis of the hand, hip, and knee. Arthritis Care Res 2012;64(4):465–74.
44. National Collaborating Centre for Chronic Conditions. Osteoarthritis: care and management. London: National Institute for Health and Clinical Excellence (NICE); 2014.
45. Physician Summary. Non-Surgical Treatment of Osteoarthritis of the Knee. OARSI. 2014. Available at: https://www.oarsi.org/education/oarsi-guidelines. Accessed November 9, 2019.
46. Drago S, Imboden R, Schlatter P, et al. Pharmacokinetics of transdermal etofenamate and diclofenac in healthy volunteers. Basic Clin Pharmacol Toxicol 2017;121:423–9.
47. Therapeutic Goods Administration. Safety review of diclofenac. Canberra: Australian Government Department of Health; 2014. Available at: https://www.tga.gov.au/safety-review-diclofenac. Accessed November 9, 2019.
48. Manvelian G, Daniels S, Gibofsky A. The pharmacokinetic parameters of a single dose of a novel nano-formulated, lower-dose oral diclofenac. Postgrad Med 2012;124(1):117–23.
49. Manvelian G, Daniels S, Altman R. A phase I study evaluating the pharmacokinetic profile of a novel, proprietary, nano-formulated, lower-dose oral indomethacin. Postgrad Med 2012;124(4):197–205.
50. Drugs@FDA. Ketorolac [Drug Label]. 2014. Available at: https://www.accessdata.fda.gov/drugsatfda_docs/label/2014/074802s038lbl.pdf. Accessed November 9, 2019.
51. Strom B, Berlin J, Kinman J, et al. Parenteral ketorolac and risk of gastrointestinal and operative site bleeding. A postmarketing surveillance study. JAMA 1996;275(5):376–82.
52. Drugs@FDA. SPRIX [Drug Label]. 2018. Available at: https://www.accessdata.fda.gov/drugsatfda_docs/label/2018/022382s018lbl.pdf. Accessed November 9, 2019.
53. Drugs@FDA. Caldolor [Drug Label]. 2019. Available at: https://www.accessdata.fda.gov/drugsatfda_docs/label/2019/022348s014lbl.pdf. Accessed November 9, 2019.
54. RECRO Pharma Press Release. FDA grants appeal to recro pharma for IV meloxicam new drug application 2019. Available at: https://ir.recropharma.com/press-releases/detail/147/fda-grants-appeal-to-recro-pharma-for-iv-meloxicam-new-drug. Accessed November 9, 2019.

Topical Analgesics

Steven Stanos, DO

KEYWORDS

- Topical analgesics • Topical NSAIDs • Nonsteroidal anti-inflammatory drugs
- Osteoarthritis guidelines • Neuropathic pain guidelines

KEY POINTS

- Topical analgesics include a wide range of compounds used for a variety of acute and chronic pain conditions, including pain related to osteoarthritis, musculoskeletal strains, and strains; muscle injuries; and neuropathic pain conditions, such as diabetic and HIV-related neuropathies, postherpetic neuralgia, and complex regional pain syndrome. Many over-the-counter topical heat and cold products also are available for daily use for soft tissue pain.
- Advancements in formulation technology have helped and will continue to contribute to develop medications that provide better penetration through the relatively impermeable skin to improve absorption to targeted tissues.
- Treatment guidelines from US and international specialty organizations have recommended greater use of topical analgesics for specific conditions due to their improved efficacy and relatively safer safety profile, helping to make topical analgesics a more valuable tool for a patient-centered treatment program that may include nonpharmacologic and pharmacologic interventions.

INTRODUCTION

Topical analgesics include a growing area of diverse prescription and over-the-counter (OTC) formulations. In 2000, topical medications for pain accounted for 6% of the US analgesic market.[1] Of the $17.8 billion spent annually on pain medications in the United States in 2007, $1.9 billion was accounted for by analgesics/nonsteroidal anti-inflammatory drugs (NSAIDs), $3.6 billion for opioids, and $12.3 billion for adjuvants.[2] Approximately 9% of the adjuvant class (antidepressants, anticonvulsants, antirheumatics, muscle relaxants, topical products, and corticosteroids) included spending for topical products. Side effect and adverse events from oral medications, including NSAID-related gastrointestinal and cardiac effects, central nervous system changes (ie cognitive impairment, dizziness) and other end-organ effects including blood pressure changes, limb swelling, and somnolence sometimes seen with the use of antidepressants, anticonvulsants, and muscle relaxers, and opioid related adverse effects and morbidities (ie constipation, cognitive impairment, misuse, abuse, dependence, and addiction), provide topical preparations as a relatively safer alternative for patients.[3,4] Because topical analgesics target peripheral tissues via direct

Swedish Pain Services, 600 Broadway, Suite #530, Seattle, WA 98112, USA
E-mail address: Steven.Stanos@swedish.org

Phys Med Rehabil Clin N Am 31 (2020) 233–244
https://doi.org/10.1016/j.pmr.2020.02.002
1047-9651/20/© 2020 Elsevier Inc. All rights reserved.

application over a painful or effected site, external delivery of the medication focally may provide greater pharmacologic effect at superficial structures, including ligaments, bursa, and joints, with less systemic effects than their oral counterparts. This article reviews topical drug delivery pharmacology and drug delivery principles and formulations for various conditions, including musculoskeletal and soft tissue disorders and agents used for neuropathic pain.

CLINICAL USE OF TOPICAL ANALGESICS: TARGETING MECHANISMS

Topical analgesics remain a growing area of interest and of scientific study for several acute and chronic pain conditions, including musculoskeletal pain, such as ligamentous strains and muscle strains, and neuropathic pain, including diabetic peripheral neuropathy, focal neuropathies, HIV-related neuropathy, complex regional pain syndrome, and postherpetic neuralgia. NSAIDs include a diverse group of agents used for systemic and local treatment of painful conditions. The initial understanding was that the mechanism of action was inhibiting the cyclooxygenase (COX) enzyme, a key enzyme in prostaglandin synthesis. Prostaglandins are hormone-like lipid compounds with multiple physiologic effects, including regulation of inflammation, pain sensitization, and platelet aggregation. There are 2 isoforms of COX: COX-1, the constitutive isoform, with primarily protective effects, and COX-2, the inducible isoform, expressed increasingly during inflammatory response.[5] Neuropathic pain targets for the heterogeneous groups of conditions can be best conceptualized by targeting clinical manifestations, including spontaneous symptoms like paresthesias and superficial skin pain; negative sensory symptoms, including hypoesthesia and hypoalgesia; and positive sensory symptoms, including mechanical allodynia, static allodynia, hyperalgesia, and hot or cold allodynia.[6] Targets include transduction, propagation, and transmission of nociceptors in the periphery by various inflammatory and noninflammatory mediators, cytokines, calcium-dependent cascades, sodium channels, and interaction with a family of heat receptors, the transient receptor potential family of ion channels. Transient receptor potentials are selective for calcium and magnesium, activated by multiple mechanisms (eg, heat, acid, inflammatory mediators, and cannabinoids).[7,8]

BENEFITS AND LIMITATIONS OF CUTANEOUS DELIVERY

The terms, *topical* and *transdermal*, although sometimes used interchangeably, are distinct delivery concepts. Although both topical delivery and transdermal delivery involve the passage of a medication across the skin, topical agents target soft tissues and peripheral nerves directly beneath the skin, using various vehicles to help to deliver the medication passively across the stratum corneum, the epidermis, the dermal layer, adipose, and deeper soft tissue structures such as the joint capsule, ligaments, tendons, and muscle. Transdermal delivery involves the passage of medication by percutaneous absorption, either by active delivery such as physical disruption of the stratum corneum or by the additional use of an external forces or modalities (heat, vehicles) to drive medication deeper in order to achieve stable systemic serum levels of the active drug. Transdermal patches or systems are applied away from the site of injury typically on the chest, arm, or abdomen.[9] Medication classes for transdermal delivery includes nicotine, fentanyl, buprenorphine, estrogen hormone replacement, birth control medications, scopolamine (motion sickness), and rotigotine (Parkinson Disease). Topical formulations are available as solutions, sprays, creams, foams, gels, patches (or plasters), and ointments.[10] Topical formulations include a wide range of agents including NSAIDs, capsaicin, anesthetics (lidocaine), and less commonly used rubefacients and salicylates. Rubefacients, such as menthol and methyl salicylate, produce skin redness. Salicylates, such as aspirin, magnesium, and sodium salicylate, were originally proposed to act as counter-irritants.

The benefits of topical and transdermal delivery include bypass of first-pass metabolism, fewer peaks and troughs compared with oral absorption, direct access to target tissues, and ease of use. Limitations for cutaneous delivery include diffusion challenges across a relatively resistant stratum corneum to molecules less than 500 Da, need for agents to have both aqueous and lipid solubility to enhance penetration, patient variability in permeability of the skin, and local skin irritation and other skin adverse effects.

PHARMACOLOGIC CONSIDERATIONS FOR TOPICAL AGENTS

Depth of penetration is important to the success of clinical application. Pharmacokinetic data of topical NSAIDs demonstrated peak plasma levels less than 10% of concentrations from oral administration, with a range of 0.2% to 8.0%.[11] A basic concept for topical formulations to be effective is that the formulation must penetrate the relatively impermeable skin barriers. Penetration below lower levels of the skin allows absorption into vascular structures and deeper areas where inflammation may be the target. A balance between lipid and aqueous solubility is necessary to maximize permeability. Additional enhancers that help drive medications across the skin have been developed and are under study including more traditional use of iontophoresis for NSAID delivery, various penetration enhancers (liposomes, nanocarriers, lecithin organogels), nanosystems such as micoremulsions and nanoemulsions, nanoparticles, flexible vesicles, and emulsions that provide lower particle size, and potentially improved thermodynamic stability. Lecithin organogels, composed of hydrated phospholipids and organic liquids, are commonly used in compounded formulations and include lecithin, pluronic gel, and isopropyl palmitate.[12] An ideal topical agent has a low molecular weight and both hydrophobic features to transverse the stratum corneum and hydrophilic properties to better penetrate the relatively aqueous epidermis.[13] Advancements in novel compounds currently in development include nanosystems, which enhance skin permeation, such as microemulsions, nanoemulsions, nanoparticles, and lipid carriers; and flexible vesicles, which help improve solubility and bioavailability. The emulsion advantages include lower particle size, transparent and fluid texture, and stable thermodynamic stability.[14,15]

Penetration into deeper tissues beneath the stratum corneum may vary and depend not only on depth but also on type of tissue. Classic penetration studies of NSAIDs showed significant concentration levels in subcutaneous and muscle of oral ibuprofen, 800 mg, versus 5% ibuprofen gel, 16 g. Probes inserted approximately 30 mm into the muscle found average values 3-times greater by oral versus topical application but 22.5-fold greater concentrations in the dermis. Other studies have demonstrated significantly greater local absorption in the periarticular structures of the joint with topical delivery of an NSAID. A study of ketoprofen patch compared to oral ketoprofen 50 mg demonstrated a 20-30 times greater concentration in the cartilage and meniscus of the knee as compared to 60-70% of concentrations in the synovium as compared to serum levels. The authors proposed that the relatively avascular cartilage and meniscus may act as a drug reservoir.[16]

SAFETY CONCERN: PHOTOSENSITIVITY

Although topical delivery of medications assumes a relatively greater safety profile, a number of agents may rarely cause mild to severe photosensitivity-like reactions. These agents include some antifungal agents, antiseptic drugs, ultraviolet radiation-blocking agents (sun tan oils and gels), in addition to some NSAIDs. Most NSAIDs as a class are photoreactive and may cause a photoallergic contact dermatitis. Case reports include rare but severe photosensitivity reactions most commonly with ketoprofen, followed by piroxicam and diclofenac.[17,18] Interestingly, 95 of the 342 topical products approved in the United States are noted to be stored in light protective packaging.[19]

CLINICAL USE OF TOPICAL ANALGESICS: SHIFTING EVIDENCE SUPPORTING GREATER USE
Update on Recent Guidelines

Controversy in the past 20 years related to adverse events of NSAIDs and selective COX-2 inhibitors and more recent challenges related to potential harm related to acute and chronic opioid use with improvements in topical delivery mechanisms and formulations have helped elevate guidelines and best practices favoring greater topical analgesic use.[20] Several US and international treatment guidelines include updated evidence related to effectiveness of topical analgesics primarily for osteoarthritis (OA) and neuropathic pain conditions. The most comprehensive Cochrane Library review of topical NSAIDs for chronic musculoskeletal pain was published in 2016 and included 10,631 participant in 39 studies.[21] Topical diclofenac and topical ketoprofen provided good levels of pain relief beyond carrier in OA (mostly from studies in knee OA) for a minority of people (10% greater than placebo) with no evidence for other chronic pain conditions. At least some of the placebo effects in longer studies were suggested to be derived from effects by the NSAID carrier. The following is an overview of recommendations from various specialty groups related to recommendations specific for topical analgesics and contains brief mentions of related medications (acetaminophen, opioids, oral NSAIDs, and tramadol) and interventions (passive modalities and acupuncture) commonly used in conjunction with topical therapies or as part of previous step therapy protocols.

Update on Neuropathic Pain Guidelines

The American Academy of Orthopaedic Surgeons clinical practice guideline, "Treatment of Osteoarthrosis of the Knee," 2nd edition (2013),[22] includes strong recommendations for oral and topical NSAIDs (based on studies on eltenac [similar to diclofenac] and ketoprofen) or tramadol for patients with symptomatic OA of the knee; they are unable to recommend for or against acetaminophen (downgraded from moderate to inconclusive evidence), opioids, or pain patches. The literature review found no relevant studies meeting inclusion criteria on opioids or pain patches for knee OA.[22]

The Osteoarthritis Research Society International (OARSI) 2014[23] guideline for treatment of adults with knee OA supports topical NSAIDs use as appropriate for all patients with knee-only OA and are safer and better tolerated compared with oral NSAIDs. Due to safety concerns about toxicity, acetaminophen was given a recommendation of uncertain. Oral and transdermal opioids with uncertain recommendations and glucosamine and chondroitin were found to be not appropriate for patients.[23]

The National Institute of Health and Care Excellence (NICE) guideline for the treatment of OA[24] recommend topical NSAIDs as second-line after first-line interventions (rest, patient education, and weight loss) due to their clinical efficacy and relative safety profile compared with traditional NSAIDs, COX-2 inhibitors, intra-articular steroid injections, therapy, and surgical interventions.

The European League Against Rheumatism (EULAR)[25] guideline recommends "local treatments to systemic treatments, especially for mild to moderate pain and when only a few joints are affected." Topical NSAIDs and capsaicin are effective and safe treatments for hand OA.

In the American College of Rheumatology/Arthritis Foundation "Guideline for the Management of Osteoarthritis of the Hand, Hip, and Knee"[26] (2020), the comprehensive guideline lays out a wide range of treatment options without the typical algorithmic, hierarchy, or stepwise recommendations classically used in most previous recommendations. The recommendations include strong recommendations for nondrug interventions and a patient-centered approach focusing on patient-level factors and emphasizing comprehensive management, including consideration of disease severity, personal beliefs, access to care, and surgical and injury history. The guidelines also advise considering an individual patient's overall well-being and perception of pain and function, mood, altered sleep, stress levels, and coping measures. A strong emphasis was placed on behavioral medicine and education and mind-body and physical approaches, including aerobic exercise, strengthening, aquatic exercise and weight loss, and multidisciplinary approaches (self-management programs). The guideline also includes strong recommendations against specific interventions such as transcutaneous electrical nerve stimulation (TENS) and conditionally recommends against the use of modified shoes, pulsed vibration therapy, wedged insoles, and massage and manual therapy for hip or knee OA. Topical NSAIDs were strongly recommended for knee pain and conditionally recommended for hand OA. Topical capsaicin is conditionally recommended for knee pain. Chondroitin is conditionally recommended for hand OA. Other oral medications (acetaminophen, tramadol, and duloxetine) are conditionally recommended for hand, knee, and hip OA (**Fig. 1**).

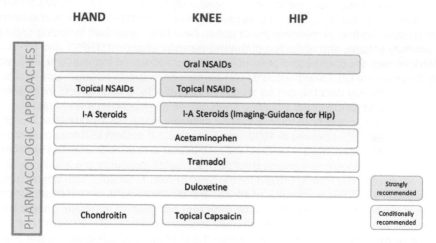

Fig. 1. Recommended therapies for the management of OA. (*Modified from* Kolasinski SL, Neogi T, Hochberg MC, et al. 2019 American college of rheumatology/arthritis foundation guideline for the management of osteoarthritis of the hand, hip, and knee. Arthritis Rheumatol. 2020; 72(2):220-233; with permission.)

TOPICAL AGENTS
Topical NSAIDs

A number of prescription strength topical NSAIDs are available worldwide and include gels, patches, solutions and compounds primarily including diclofenac, ibuprofen, ketoprofen, eltenac, felbinac and piroxicam.[27] Safety studies have examined the adverse effects of topical NSAIDs as compared to oral use including the use of these products in older patients and those with medical comorbidities demonstrating similar and low rates of adverse events in older patients and those with comorbid hypertension, diabetes, cerebrovascular and cardiovascular disease.[28,29] Despite the evidence supporting a greater safety profile as compared to oral NSAIDs, topical NSAIDs, including prescription and over-the counter products, all carry the same black-box warnings related to potential NSAID-related risks for cardiovascular, renal, and gastrointestinal events.

In the US all of the 4 approved FDA products are diclofenac-based formulations. Diclofenac is an acetic acid derivative similar to indomethacin and ketorolac. Diclofenac has a relatively rapid absorption and short half-life orally and is usually supplied in various salts such as diclofenac sodium or diclofenac epolamine. Current FDA approved NSAIDs in the US are diclofenac-based products. Indications spine a range of musculoskeletal conditions including for the treatment of superficial joint OA (hands, knees) for diclofenac gel, sprains and strains for diclofenac epolamine patch, and to treat signs and symptoms associated with knee osteoarthritis (diclofenac sodium solution 1.5% and a more viscous solution as a 2% foam) (**Table 1**). Both diclofenac 1.5% vs 1% foam contain dimethyl sulfoxide (DMSO) which may be provide an additional vehicle to deliver the solution deeper into the superficial layers beneath the relatively impermeable stratum corneum.

Efficacy and safety data is available for other topical NSAIDs, including ketoprofen, and ibuprofen in the form of various gels, solutions, and patches but these products are currently not FDA approved for use in the US.[30,31]

Topical Lidocaine

Lidocaine is an amide anesthetic the non-selectively blocks sodium channels on sensory afferents including $A\delta$ and c-fibers causing reduced ectopic discharge and signal propagation. Additional mechanisms of action have been proposed including anti-inflammatory actions, and activation of thermo-receptor channels (TRPV1 and TRPA1).

Various over-the counter and prescription strength lidocaine formulations are available for use in the US. Over-the counter preparations are approved under less rigorous safety and efficacy data but can be an option for patients. OTC products include 4% patch formulations marketed including such names as Aspercreme and Salonpas.

Prescription lidocaine products presently available in the US include lidocaine 5% patch (Lidoderm)[32] approved in 1999, and lidocaine 1.8 system (ZTlido) approved in 2018.[33] Generic lidocaine 5% patches are also available in the US. Both the Lidoderm 5% patch and lidocaine 1.8% system (ZTlido) patch products are similar in size (10 × 14 cm) and are FDA approved for the relief of pain associated with postherpetic neuralgia (PHN).[34] The percentage of lidocaine in these products are not based on potency of the lidocaine anesthetic but by milligram per gram of adhesive. Thus a lidocaine 5% lidocaine patch (Lidoderm patch) is approximately 700 mg and 14 gm by weight or 5% and lidocaine topical system 1.8% (ZTlido) which is 36 mg per 2 gm by weight is 1.8%. Lidocaine topical system 1.8% is a nonaqueous based patch as compared to lidocaine 5% patch (hydrogel patch system) and thus lighter in weight, as well as has a lower drug load by weight (36 mg vs 700 mg in the lidoderm 5% patch) to achieve same effects, which both may contribute to greater levels of adhesiveness in trials used for FDA approval.

Lidocaine patches are recommended as 1st line or 2nd line for neuropathic pain including PHN by various published neuropathic pain guidelines (**Table 2**).[35–37]

Baron and colleagues[38] studied lidocaine 5% patch use compared to oral anticonvulsant, pregabalin (FDA approved for PHN) in an open-label study of patients with PHN and diabetic peripheral neuropathy (DPN). The primary endpoint was response rate at 4 weeks (average reduction over the last three days from baseline or > or == 2 point or an absolute value of < or = 4 points on the 11-point Numerical Rating Scale [NRS-3]). Sixty six percent of patient treated with lidocaine 5% patch and 61% of those receiving pregabalin were

Table 1
US FDA approved NSAIDs for topical use

Agent (Brand Name)	Formulation	Dosing Instructions	Indication
Diclofenac Sodium solution 1.5% w/w(Pennsaid)	1.5% solution (with DMSO 45.5% w/w/); 1 mL solution = 16.05 mg of diclofenac sodium	40 drops applied to the knee four times daily or 50 drops to the knee 3 times per day at evenly spaced intervals. Apply 10 drops at a time.	To treat signs and symptoms associated with knee osteoarthritis
Diclofenac sodium topical solution 2% w/w (Pennsaid)	2% Solution (Foam) with DMSO 45.5% w/w/; 1 gm solution = 20 mg diclofenac sodium	Apply 2 pump actuations on each painful knee, 2 times a day (40 mg = 2 pumps)	For the relief of pain of OA joints amenable to topical treatment, such as the knees and hands
Diclofenac sodium gel 1% (Voltaren Gel)	Gel	Adults: 4 g for each knee, ankle, or foot 4 times per day to any 1 affected joint of the lower extremities. Do not exceed more than 16 g daily to any one affected lower extremity joint of the lower extremities. Apply 2 g for each elbow, wrist, or hand 4 times per day. Do not apply more than 8 g daily to any 1 affected upper extremity joint. Do not exceed a total dose of 32 g per day over all affected joints	For relief of pain of OA of joints amenable to topical treatment, such as the knees and those of the hands
Diclofenac epolamine 1.3% patch (Flector)	Topical system 1.3% patch; 180 mg of diclofenac epolamine (13 mg of diclofenac epolamine per gram of adhesive)	Apply 1 patch to painful area twice daily	For the topical treatment of acute pain due to minor strains, sprains, and contusions in adults and pediatric patients 6 y and older

Abbreviation: DMSO, dimethyl sulfoxide.

considered positive responders while responder rates were similar in subjects with DPN. Both lidocaine patch and pregabalin subjects showed reductions in allodynia. Lidocaine 5% patch showed greater improvements in quality of life in PHN and DPN.

Off-label use of Lidoderm patches are common and include for the use of other peripheral nerve entrapment neuropathies and diabatic neuropathy although efficacy and study sizes vary.[39,40] Two open- label studies of 20 and 100 patients, respectively, examined lidocaine 5% patch us in patients with osteoarthritis of the knee demonstrating statistically significant improvements in pain and neuropathic pain scale

Table 2
Topical agents for neuropathic pain: guideline recommendations

	Dose	NeuPSIG	EFNS
Lidocaine patch • Lidocaine 5% patch (Lidoderm Patch) • Lidocaine 1.8% system (ZTlido)	Apply only once for up to 12 h within a 24 h period (maximum of 3) to intact skin	2nd line peripheral neuropathic pain; 1st line when there are concerns with side effects or safety of first line treatments, particularly in frail and elderly patients	1st line PHN, especially the elderly if there are concerns regarding CNS side effects
Capsaicin cream			2nd line PHN
Capsaicin 8% patch (Qutenza®)	1 or 4 patches to the painful area for 30 min (feet) or 60 min (other areas of the body excluding above the neck) every 3 mo	2nd line peripheral NP	2nd line painful HIV neuropathies or PHN

Abbreviations: EFNS, European Federation of Neurological Societies; HIV, human immunodeficiency virus; NeuPSIG, Special Interest Group on Neuropathic Pain; NP, neuropathic pain.
Data from Refs.[35–37]

scores although the authors recommended further larger randomized controlled trials were needed.[41,42] The reader is referred to a recent comprehensive review of current and developing lidocaine formulations.[43]

Capsaicinoids: Capsaicin-Based Gels and Patches

Capsaicin is a naturally occurring spicy and pungent molecule found in various foods (s.a. bell peppers, jalapeno, tai pepper, and habanero) and a range of household products. Capsaicin, a capsaicinoid, is a highly selective agonist of the TRPV1 receptors found on C fibers and Aδ fibers, and can be activated by heat (>43°C), pH changes (<6.0), and endogenous lipids leading to nerve depolarization causing local burning, stinging, and itching sensations. Clinical use of capsaicin topically in the 1980s led to cloning and understanding or vanilloid receptors and further research relating to temperature receptors including the discovery of the transient receptor potential (TRP) family of ion channels.[44] Early work with the transient receptor potential vanilloid receptor 1 (TRPV1) identified by cloning of capsaicin has contributed to the advancement of agonist-based therapies. TRPV1 is expressed in C-fibers and may interact with morphine and cannabinoids.[45] Although the initial understanding of capsaicin induced pain relief in the 1980's focused on the impact of substance P depletion and neurogenic inflammation which follows after repeated applications, this mechanism is now thought to be a transient or acute phenomena. Additional mechanisms are thought to underlie what is now referred to as capsaicin-induced "defunctionalization" including inactivation of voltage-gated Na channels, desensitization of plasma membrane TRPV1 receptors, overwhelming effects of intracellular Ca^{++} entering the cell, activation of calcium-dependent proteases and cytoskeleton breakdown.[46]

A number of over-the-counter and prescription capsaicin products are available and are easily classified as low-concentration (<1%) OTCs or high concentration products. Low-concentration preparations include 0.025%, 0.075%, and 0.1% OTC creams and high concentration prescription strength formulation of 8% capsaicin in a patch system (Qutenza®). Ultra-potent products, such as resiniferatoxin, are used for bladder installation for interstitial cystitis and other medical conditions.

Both low-concentration preparations are used off label for neuropathic pain (PHN and DPN) and musculoskeletal conditions, including osteoarthritis and muscle pain. Recommended dosing is application to the effected skin area 3 to 4 times per day for at least 4 to 6 weeks. Patients should wash their hand with soap and water after application to avoid contamination and irritation to the eyes or face. An early meta-analysis of capsaicin cream for the treatment of DPN, osteoarthritis and PHN found evidence for greater pain relief in DPN and OA versus placebo, less convincing evidence for PHN, and concern regarding challenges of blinding subjects.[47] Widespread use of capsaicin creams has been limited by poor efficacy, patient tolerability and compliance in that patients had to apply the pungent creams two to three times per day causing a burning sensation in order to produce a pharmacologic desensitization of the skin in order to achieve longer term pain relief by functionally desensitizing the target tissue.[48] Kulkantrokorn and colleagues[49] studied 0.025% OTC capsaicin gel for patients with DPN demonstrating no benefit versus placebo. Capsaicin patches or plasters, as described outside of the US, have shown some efficacy in low back pain. Frerick and colleagues[50] reported on the use of "capsicum" plaster for non-specific low back pain, in a double-blind, placebo-controlled study. After 3 weeks subjects treated with capsicum reported a 42% reduction in compound pain score versus 31% reduction in the placebo group.

Capsaicin 8% (Qutenza®) was approved in 2009 for the treatment of neuropathic pain associated with PHN in the US and in Europe for peripheral neuropathic pain in non-diabetic adults.[51] In deference to the low dose formulations that are limited by poor patient compliance and need for repeat dosing, capsaicin 8% is a single application done under supervision of a physician, usually in an outpatient setting. The skin are involved is prepped with high dose lidocaine to anesthetize the skin prior to the careful placement of the product over the involved are for 30 to 60 min. The skin is then carefully cleaned to eliminate any residual capsaicin on the skin. Patch application can be repeated every 3 months. Capsaicin 8% is FDA approved for PHN. Capsaicin patch 8% applied to the skin for 60 minutes was more effective than a low concentration patch (0.04%) in a 3 month trial.[52]

SUMMARY

Topical analgesics include a wide range of formulations involved in the treatment of both musculoskeletal and neuropathic pain conditions. Advancements in formulation technology has evolved and potentially may lead to improved delivery of medication deeper into the target tissues. Topical analgesics, due to their superficial effects, have demonstrated a significant safety profile due to minimal systemic absorption as compared to their oral or transdermal counterparts.

Treatment guidelines from various scientific societies and specialty groups recommend an expanding use of these topical analgesics earlier in the treatment regimen. An understanding and elucidation of thermal receptors from the use of capsaicin in the early 1980s contributed to the development of topical capsaicinoids for the treatment of neuropathic pain and some evidence for musculoskeletal conditions.

This Clinics overview included a discussion of many of the topical formulations FDA approved in the US, but is in no means a complete one. Additional products, many formulated from compounding pharmacies, and the growing number of combination OTC products, represent a additional options for patients, although the general evidence from the medical literature has not supported the efficacy of compounded products compared to placebo.[53] Combination topical analgesics for a number of musculoskeletal and neuropathic pain conditions including the use of ketamine, amitriptyline, and gabapentin have been published, mostly involving smaller groups of patients. The reader is referred to additional topical analgesic reviews to supplement this article.[54–56]

DISCLOSURE

Pfizer, Salix, and Sanofi: consultant; Scilex: consultant and promotional speaking for lidocaine topical 1.8% (ZTlido).

REFERENCES

1. Datamonitor. United States-analgesics. New York NY. Reference code 72-751. Available at: www.datamonitor.com. Accessed January 28, 2007.
2. Rasu RS, Vouthy K, Crowl A, et al. Cost of pain medication to treat adult patients with nonmalignant chronic pain in the United States. J Manag Care Pharm 2014;20:921–8.
3. Conaghan PG. A turbulent decade for NSAIDs: Update on current concepts of classification, epidemiology, comparative efficacy, and toxicity. Rheumatol Int 2012;32(6):1491–502.
4. Scanzello CR, Moskowitz NK, Gibofsky A. The post-NSAID era: what to use now for pharmacologic treatment of pain and inflammation in osteoarthritis. Curr Rheumatol Rep 2008;10:49–56.
5. Dubois RN, Abramson SB, Crofford L, et al. Cycloxygenase in biology and disease. FASEB J 1998;1063–73.
6. Baron R. Neuropathic pain: diagnosis, pathophysiological mechanisms, and treatment. Lancet Neurol 2010;9:807–19.
7. Knotkova H, Pappagallo M, Szallasi A. Capsaicin (TRPV1 Agonist) therapy for pain relief farewell or revival? Clin J Pain 2008;24:142–54.
8. Szallasi A, Blumberg P. Vanilloid (capsaicin) receptors and mechanisms. Pharmacol Res 1989;2:159–211.
9. Watkinson EC, Kearney MC, Quinn HL, et al. Future of the transdermal drug delivery market – have we barely touched the surface? Expert Opin Drug Deliv 2016;13(4):523–32.
10. Stanos SP. Topical agents for the management of musculoskeletal pain. J Pain Symptom Manage 2007;33:342–55.
11. Heyneman CA, Lawless-Liday C, Wall GC. Oral versus topical NSAIDs in rheumatic diseases: a comparison. Drugs 2000;60(3):555–74.
12. Franckum J, Ramsay D, Das NG, et al. Pluronic lecithin organogel for local delivery of anti-inflammatory drugs. Int J Pharm Compd 2004;8(2):101–5.
13. Vaile JH, Davis P. Topical NSAIDs for musculoskeletal conditions. A review of the literature. Drugs 1998;56(5):783–99.
14. Christofori C, Ponto T, Abd E, et al. Topical nano and microemulsions for skin delivery. Pharmaceutics 2017;9:37.
15. Tegeder I, Muth-Selbach U, Lotsch J, et al. Application of microdialysis for the determination of muscle and subcutaneous tissue concentrations after oral and topical ibuprofen administration. Clin Pharmacol Ther 1999;65(4):357–68.
16. Rolf C, Engstrom B, Beauchard C, et al. Intra-articular absorption and distribution of ketoprofen after topical plaster application and oral intake in 100 patients undergoing knee arthroscopy. Rheumatology (Oxford) 1999;38(6):564–7.
17. Rindo T, Oiso N, Yamadori Y, et al. Photoallergic contact dermatitis due to ketoprofen and hydrogenated rosin glycerol ester. Case Rep Dermatol 2010;2:36–9.
18. Matthieu L, Meuleman L, Hecke EV, et al. Contact and photocontact allergy to ketoprofen. The Belgian experience. Contact Dermatitis 2004;50:238–41.
19. Kryczyk-Poprawa A, Kwiecien A, Opoka W. Photostability of topical agents applied to the skin: a review. Pharmaceutics 2020;12:10.
20. Brown M, Martin GP, Jonas SA, et al. Dermal and transdermal drug delivery systems: current and future prospects. Drug Deliv 2006;13(3):175–87.

21. Denny S, Conaghan P, Da Silva JA, et al. Topical NSAIDs for chronic musculo-skeletal pain in adults. Cochrane Database Syst Rev 2016;(4):CD007400.
22. American Academy of Orthopaedic Surgeons. Treatment of osteoarthritis of the knee. Evidence-based guideline. 2nd edition. Rosemont (IL): 2013.
23. OARSI Reference.
24. National Institute for Health and Clinical Excellence (NICE). CG 59 Osteoarthritis: the care and management of osteoarthritis in adults. London: NICE; 2008. Available at: www.nice.org.uk/GG059. Accessed September, 2008.
25. Zhang, et al. (FIX) European league against rheumatism. Ann Rheum Dis 2007;66:3.
26. Kolasinski S, Neogi T, Hochberg M, et al. 2019 American College of Rheumatology/Arthritis Foundation guideline for the management of osteoarthritis of the hand, hip, and knee. Arthritis Care Res 2020;72(2):149–62.
27. Altman RD, Barthel HR. Topical therapies for osteoarthritis. Drugs 2017;71(10):1259–79.
28. Baraf HS, Gold M, Petruschke R, et al. Tolerability of topical diclofenac sodium 1% gel for osteoarthritis in seniors and patients with comorbidities. Am J Geriatr Pharmacother 2011;10(1):47–60.
29. Baraf HS, Gloth FM, Barthel HR, et al. Safety and efficacy of topical diclofenac sodium gel for knee osteoarthritis in elderly and younger patients: pooled data from three randomized, double-blind, parallel-group, placebo-controlled, multi-centre trials. Drugs Aging 2011;28:27–40.
30. Sardana V, Burzynski J, Zaizal P. Safety and efficacy of topical ketoprofen in transfersome gel in knee osteoarthritis: a systematic review. Musculoskeletal Care 2017;15:114–21.
31. Lewis F, Connolly MP, Bhatt A. A pharmacokinetic study of an ibuprofen topical patch in healthy male and female adult volunteers. Clin Pharmacol Drug Dev 2018;7(7):684–91.
32. Endo Pharmaceuticals Inc. Malvern, PA. LIDODERM PatchÒ Prescribing Information. January, 2015.
33. Scilex Pharmaceuticals. ZTLidoÔ Prescribing Information. 2018, April.
34. Rowbotham MC, Davies PS, Verkempinck C, et al. Lidocaine patch: double-blind controlled study of a new treatment method for post-herpetic neuralgia. Pain 1996;65:39–44.
35. Sommer C, Cruccu G. Topical treatment of peripheral neuropathic pain: applying the evidence. J Pain Symptom Manage 2017;53:614–29.
36. Finnerup NB, Attal N, Haroutounian S, et al. Pharmacotherapy for neuropathic pain in adults: a systematic review and meta-analysis. Lancet Neurol 2015;2:162–73. NeuPSIG.
37. Attal N, Cruccu G, Baron R, et al EFNS guidelines on the pharmacological treatment of neuropathic pain: 2010 revision. Eur J Neurol 2010;17:113–1123. EFNS.
38. Baron R, Mayoral V, Leijon G, et al. 5% lidocaine medicated plaster versus pregabalin in post-herpetic neuralgia and diabetic polyneuropathy: an open-label, non-inferiority two-stage RCT study. Curr Med Res Opin 2009;25(7):1663–76.
39. Meier T, Wasner T, Faust M, et al. Efficacy of lidocaine patch 5% in the treatment of focal peripheral neuropathic pain syndromes: a randomized, double-blind, placebo-controlled study. Pain 2003;106:151–8.
40. Barbano RL, Hermann DN, Hart-Gouleau S, et al. Effectiveness, tolerability, and impact on quality of life of the 5% lidocaine patch in diabetic polyneuropathy. Arch Neurol 2004;61:914–8.
41. Galer BS, Sheldon E, Patel N, et al. Topical lidocaine patch 5% may target a novel underling pain mechanism in osteoarthritis. Curr Med Res Opin 2004;20(9):1455–8.

42. Gammaitoni AR, Galer BS, Onawola R, et al. Lidocaine patch 5% and its positive impact on pain qualities in osteoarthritis: results of a pilot 2-week, open-label study using the Neuropathic pain scale. Curr Med Res Opin 2004;20(Suppl 2):S13–9.
43. Gudin J, Nalamachu S. Utility of lidocaine as a topical analgesic and improvements in patch delivery systems. Postgrad Med 2020;132(1):28–36.
44. Szallasi A, Blumberg P. Vanilloid (capsaicin) receptors and mechanisms. Pharmacol Res 1989;2:159–211.
45. Knotkova H, Pappagallo M, Szallasi A. Capsaicin (TRPV1 Agonist) therapy for pain relief farewell or revival? Clin J Pain 2008;24:142–54.
46. Anand P, Bley K. Topical capsaicin for pain management: therapeutic potential and mechanisms of action of the new high-concentration capsaicin 8% patch. Br J Anaesth 2011;107(4):490–502.
47. Zhang WY, Po A. The effectiveness of topically applied capsaicin. A meta-analysis. Eur J Clin Pharmacol 1994;46:517–22.
48. Derry S, Moore R. Topical capsaicin (low concentration) for chronic neuropathic pain in adults. Cochrane Database Syst Rev 2012;9:CD010111.
49. Kulkantrokorn K, Lorsuwansiris C, Meesawatsom P. 0.025% capsaicin gel for the treatment of painful diabetic neuropathy: a randomized, double-blind, crossover, placebo-controlled trial. Pain Pract 2013. https://doi.org/10.1111/papr.12013.
50. Frerick H, Keite W, Kuhn U, et al. Chronic low back pain with a capsicum plaster. Pain 2003;106(1–2):59–64.
51. Qutenza Prescribing Inormation. Available at: www.qutenza.com/pdfs/Qutenza_Prescribing_Information.pdf. Accessed March 5, 2020.
52. Backonja M, Wallace MS, Blonsky ER, et al. NGX-4010, a high concentration capsaicin patch, for the treatment of postherpetic neuralgia: a randomized, double-blind study. Lancet Neurol 2009;7:1106–12.
53. Brutcher RE, Kurihara C, Bicket MC, et al. Compounded topical pain creams to treat localized chronic pain: a randomized controlled trial. Ann Intern Med 2019;170(5):309–18.
54. Stanos SP. Topical agents for the management of musculoskeletal pain. J Pain Symptom Manage 2007;33:342–55.
55. Argoff CE. Topical analgesic in the management of acute and chronic pain. Mayo Clin Proc 2013;88(2):195–205.
56. Sawnok J. Topical analgesics for neuropathic pain: preclinical exploration, clinical validation, future development. Eur J Pain 2014;18:465–81.

Muscle Relaxants for Acute and Chronic Pain

Wilson J. Chang, MD, MPH

KEYWORDS

- Low back pain • Muscle relaxants • Muscle relaxers • Spasm • Antispasmodic
- Spasticity • Antispasticity • Myofascial pain

KEY POINTS

- Types of muscle relaxants and adverse effects are examined.
- Pharmacologic indications for each type of muscle relaxant are highlighted.
- Guidance concerning appropriate utilization of muscle relaxants when treating acute and chronic low back pain is provided.

BACKGROUND

Skeletal muscle relaxants are poorly defined and understood. Conventionally defined as pharmacologic agents that are thought to produce relaxation of skeletal muscles, the various types of skeletal muscle relaxants each function in a different fashion[1-4] (**Table 1**). Little is known about the mechanism of action of several of these agents. These studies are limited in number, and most of them are based on animal models alone.[5] Furthermore, there is a lack of a consolidated source for skeletal muscle relaxants. Currently available publications are comprised mostly of US Food and Drug Administration (FDA) comparison studies that are over 30 years old.[6,7]

Skeletal muscle relaxants are also challenged by the lack of clarity in indications or diagnoses of usage. Instituted intuitively for tension-related conditions, prescribers can often confuse clinical applications for muscle spasms,[8] spasticity, or myofascial pain[9] (**Table 2**).[10] When the pathophysiology of each of these conditions differs, the ease with which skeletal muscle relaxants are prescribed can be called into question. The need to further understand clinical conditions for which these medications are prescribed becomes crucial.

PATHOPHYSIOLOGY

Basic muscle physiology will be described to better understand the regulatory systems and pathways associated with muscle activity. Muscle regulation is generally considered to act centrally or peripherally. The central nervous system (CNS) involves

Swedish Pain Services, Swedish Health System, 600 Broadway Suite 530, Seattle, WA 98122, USA
E-mail address: wilson.chang@swedish.org

Phys Med Rehabil Clin N Am 31 (2020) 245–254
https://doi.org/10.1016/j.pmr.2020.01.005

Table 1
Common skeletal muscle relaxants

	Drug	Onset	Duration	Starting Dose	Therapeutic Dose	Adverse Effects	Note
Centrally Acting	*Sedative*						
	Metaloxone	1hr	4-6 hr	400 mg TID	800 mg TID	Hemolytic anemia, headache, dz, dr, N/V	Additive effects with alcohol and CNS depressants
	Methocarbamol	30 min	N/A	500 mg QID	750 mg QID	Blurred vision, dz, dr	
	Carisoprodol	30 min	4-6 hr	350 mg TID	350 mg QID	Ataxia, withdrawal potential, dz, dr, N/V	
	Chlorzaxone	1hr	3-4 hr	250 mg QID	500 mg QID	Headache, dz, dr, N/V	
	TCA-like						
	Cyclobenzaprine	1hr	12–24 hr	5mg TID	10–20 mg TID	Dry mouth, dz, dr	Additive effects with alcohol, TCAs, and CNS depressants, seizures with tramadol and MAO-I
	GABA Agonist						
	Diazepam	30 min	variable	2 mg twice daily	5 mg 3 times daily	Ataxia, respiratory depression, hypotension, withdrawal potential	CNS depression with opioids, potentiation with barbiturates/ MAO-I
	Baclofen	3-4 d orally	variable	5 mg 3 times daily	10–20 mg 3 times daily	Slurred speech, urinary retention, constipation, dr	Short-term memory loss with antidepressants, additive effects with TCAs
		30 min IT	4-6 hr	variable	variable	Overdose/withdrawal potential	Requires slow taper because of withdrawal seizures and hallucinations

Alpha 2 Adrenergic Agonist

Drug						
Tizanidine	2 wk	variable	2mg TID	4mg TID	Paradoxic spasm/tone, dry mouth, dz, dr	Additive effects with alcohol and CNS depressants, reduced clearance with oral contraceptives. Requires slow taper
Clonidine	1 hr	24 hr	0.1 mg twice daily	0.1 mg 3 times daily	Hypotension, rebound hypertension	
Antihistamine						
Orphenadrine	1 hr	4-6 hr	100 mg twice daily	100 mg 3 times daily	Tachycardia, dry mouth, N/V	Confusion/anxiety/tremors with propoxyphene
Peripherally Acting Dantrolene	1 wk	12 hr	25 mg daily	100 mg twice daily	Tachycardia, photosensitivity, seizures	Pancytopenia with chronic use

Abbreviations: CNS, central nervous system; dr, drowsiness; dz, dizziness; GABA, gama-aminobutyric acid; IT, intrathecal; MAO-I, monoamine oxidase inhibitor; N/V, nausea/vomiting; TCA, tricyclic antidepressant.

Table 2
Comparison of spasticity, spasm, and myofascial pain

Description	Spasm	Spasticity	Myofascial Pain
Definition	Involuntary muscle contractions	Velocity-dependent increase in muscle tone caused by CNS dysfunction	Nociceptive pain derived from mechanical injury of soft tissue
Pathophysiology	Peripheral	Central	Peripheral
Etiology	Muscle sprain/injury Nerve compression	Upper motor neuron disorder/injury	Muscle sprain/tears Metabolic/ inflammatory
Symptoms	Jerks Twitch Cramps	Incessant hypertonicity/ stiffness Hyper-reflexia	Tenderness Tightness Limited range of motion
Clinical conditions	Musculoskeletal pain Mechanical dysfunction Spine-related neural impingement (radiculopathy, spinal stenosis) Fibromyalgia	Spinal cord injury Stroke Traumatic brain injury Motor neuron disease Multiple sclerosis Cerebral palsy	Myalgia Myopathic pain syndrome

a complex network of excitatory and inhibitory pathways that synapse to an inter-neuron, which in turn, makes postsynaptic connection to alpha motor neurons in the ventral horn of the spinal cord. Efferent pathway eventually synapses with the extrafusal muscle fibers, which are generally thought to control muscle contractility.[11] In contrast, intrafusal muscle fibers, which are generally thought to control muscle length through spindle structure, detect sensory inputs using the afferent pathway.[10] Such inputs include the detection of stretch. The afferent pathway synapse in the dorsal horn of the spinal cord, which serves to activate both large alpha motor neurons and small gamma motor neurons in the ventral horn. Both of these pathways synapse at extrafusal and intrafusal fibers, respectively, to exert motor influence.

The physiology of muscle regulation becomes more important when considering the indications of medication use and the co-morbidities of patients. This will be discussed further in a later section.

TYPES OF SKELETAL MUSCLE RELAXANTS
Antispasmodic Versus Antispasticity Versus Myofascial Pain

Spasticity is defined as a velocity-dependent resistance to passive movement of the affected muscles at rest. It presents as incessant increased tone, and often involves irregularity in posturing during ambulation or with noxious stimuli. Spasticity results from a centralized etiology such as stroke, cerebral palsy, or spinal cord injury among other causes. Symptoms include constant stiffness, hypertonicity, and hyper-reflexia. Antispasticity agents include baclofen, diazepam, tizanidine, and dantrolene (**Fig. 1**).

Spasm is a more generalized term that is defined as an involuntary contraction of muscles. Unlike spasticity, it can be intermixed with voluntary atonic periods. Its etiology is often peripheral because of a muscle sprain or injury but it can also stem from neuropathy of central origin. Symptoms include jerks, twitches, and cramps.

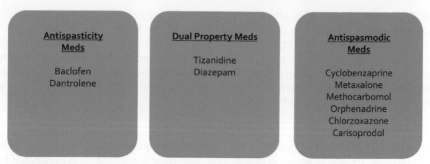

Fig. 1. List of medications with properties of antispasticity, antispasmodic, or dual functioning. (*Adapted from* Witenko C, Moorman-Li R, Motycha C, et al. Considerations for the appropriate use of skeletal muscle relaxants for the management of acute low back pain. P.T. 2014;39(6)427–435.)

Antispasmodic agents include cyclobenzaprine, carisoprodol, metaxalone, methocarbamol, orphenadrine, chlorzoxazone, diazepam, andtizanidine (see **Fig. 1**).[12]

Myofascial pain originates at the taut band of muscle. Often referred to as trigger points, these areas can be active – if painful without manipulation – or latent.[13] In contrast to an acute injury, myofascial pain is generally suggestive of a chronic state manifested in local or referred pain involving motor, sensory, and sometimes autonomic symptoms.[14] Pain related to acute or subacute mechanical injuries encompassing skeletal muscles, ligaments, labrum, and tendons is referred to musculoskeletal pain. Myofascial pain areas are often localized but can be generalized in a multifocal fashion. Painful areas are associated with tenderness, tightness, and limited range of motion. What actually constitutes a painful muscle spasms remains unclear[8] (**Table 2**).

SEDATIVE
Metaxalone

FDA approved in 1964,[15] metaxalone is a centrally acting muscle relaxant with an onset of 1 hour. Duration is 4 to 6 hours. The exact mechanism of action is unclear. Metaxalone is generally considered to be well tolerated with the exception of it being known cause of hemolytic anemia in rare cases.[16] Caution is advised with patients with hepatic or renal impairment.

Methocarbamol

FDA approved in 1964,[17] methocarbamol is available for oral, intramuscular, or intravenous use. The mechanism of action in humans is not established.[18] Methocarbamol and its metabolites are known to be excreted in the milk of dogs.[14] Complications from intravenous usage include skin sloughing and thrombophlebitis. The intravenous formulation is not recommended for patients with renal impairment.

Carisoprodol

FDA approved in 1959, carisoprodol's mechanism of action is thought to inhibit descending reticular formation in the spinal cord of animal models.[19] Carisoprodol is almost exclusively metabolized through the liver. A metabolite is meprobamate, a schedule IV substance, which is responsible for dependence. Reeves and colleagues[20,21] demonstrated that 40% of participants with a known history of substance abuse used in larger amounts than prescribed, 30% used for mood-altering effects other than pain; 20% to 30% also reported aberrant use within 3 months. Because of its dependence potential, the use of this medication has been greatly discouraged in recent times. In 2007, the European Medicines Agency recommended the suspension of marketing authorization of carisoprodol-containing products.[10] Its Committee for Medicinal Products for Human Use concluded that the risk of the medication is greater than the benefits.[10] Patients with a known history of long-term use should be tapered with goals of eventual discontinuation.

Chlorzoxazone

Chlorzoxazone is a centrally acting antispasticity medication that inhibits polysynaptic spinal reflexes. Its effectiveness is questioned, and clinical application is minimal.[22] It is known to have a short list of adverse reactions and drug interactions compared with other skeletal muscle relaxants. It should be avoided in patients with hepatic impairment.

TRICYCLIC ANTIDEPRESSANT-LIKE MEDICATIONS
Cyclobenzaprine

With a chemical structure similar to tricyclic antidepressants (TCAs), cyclobenzaprine was FDA approved in 1977.[6] It is thought to relieve muscle spasm of local origin without disrupting motor function. The mechanism of action is similar to the likes of amitriptyline, with serotonin receptors at the spinal cord or brain stem to block alpha motor neuron excitation.[23] Animal studies suggest reduced hyperactivity of skeletal muscles. Duration is 8 to 37 hours. Therapeutic doses are achieved in 3 to 4 days when plasma concentrations are greater than 4 times than single doses of the medication.[5] Borenstein and Korn[24] demonstrated symptomatic relief of acute back pain in less than 3 days of treatment; Browning and colleagues[25] demonstrated clinical efficacy most participants in the first 4 days of treatment, seemingly suggesting clinical utility in the acute phase of pain. Conversely, Leite and colleagues[26] found insufficient evidence for myofascial pain.

The adverse effect profile is similar to that of TCAs. Anticholinergic effects include dry mouth, urinary retention, constipation, and orthostasis. It is generally avoided in patients with congestive heart failure, history of myocardial infarctions, and hypermetabolic states. Concomitant use with selective serotonin reuptake inhibitors (SSRIs) can provoke serotonin syndrome.[27] Use with tramadol is known to lower the seizure threshold. There have been reported cases of hallucinations and confusion associated with possible CNS depression. This medication is not recommended for the elderly because of anticholinergic and sedative adverse effects. The American Geriatrics Society Beers Criteria label cyclobenzaprine as 1 of the skeletal muscle relaxants to avoid in elderly populations.[28]

GABA AGONIST
Diazepam

Diazepam centrally acts as a GABA agonist at the presynaptic GABA a receptors.[29] It serves to inhibit monosynaptic and polysynaptic spinal reflex pathways. The overall effect is membrane hyperpolarization and decreased neuronal firing. Diazepam has well known diverse clinical utility with a plethora of clinical effects. Depending on the prescriber's subspecialty, diazepam is used as an anxiolytic, antiepileptic, or an antispasmodic agent. What is also known about the class of benzodiazepines is their reinforcing effects as both a sedative and anxiolytic. As a result, the perceived psychiatric and psychological benefits experienced by patients allow for potential dependence and abuse. It is also worth noting that diazepam also requires a gradual taper, with a known history of chronic use because serious, sometimes fatal, withdrawal effects.

Baclofen

Baclofen centrally acts as a GABA agonist at the presynaptic GABA b receptors.[23] The influx of calcium suppresses the excitation of the presynaptic axon, which in turn, surpasses the activation of the postsynaptic receptors. This helps dampen the gamma motor neuron activation of intrafusal fibers, eventually decreasing the muscle spindle activity. The end result is inhibition of the monosynaptic and polysynaptic reflex pathways of the spine. Baclofen is also thought to reduce substance P in the spinal cord, contributing to reduction in pain. It is available in oral and intrathecal formulations. Direct introduction of medication to the cerebral spinal fluid has been proven to be effective in the treatment of some refractory cases of spasticity. Baclofen should not be stopped abruptly in patients with known history of chronic use. A slow taper is recommend to avoid withdrawal symptoms, including seizures and hallucinations.

ALPHA 2 ADRENERGIC AGONIST
Tizanidine

Tizanidine is FDA approved for treatment of muscle spasticity resulting from CNS disorders such as spinal cord injury and stroke. Although it has a similar chemical structure to clonidine, tizanidine does not share the antihypertensive effects or exert any benefit for treatment of dysautonomia.[30] Tizanidine has a short half-life, which results in frequent dosing. Studies show equivocal data for effective monotherapy treatment for muscle spasm, or myofascial pain.[31,32] There might be more support for its use in therapy for acute back pain. Dual therapy with nonsteroidal anti-inflammatory drugs (NSAIDs) has been suggested to be more effective for acute low back pain management.[33] This might be taken in consideration, as animal studies have shown antinociceptive and gastroprotective effects of tizanidine.[34] The use of tizanidine in patients with known renal impairment is cautioned. It is contraindicated in use with intravenous ciprofloxacin because of inhibition of cytochrome P450.[29]

Clonidine

Clonidine is a centrally acting alpha 2 adrenergic agonist that exerts effects at the locus ceruleus.[29] In the spinal cord, it inhibits presynaptic activity of sensory afferents. Some studies suggest it is a more effective antispasticity agent for supraspinal - brain stem or high cervical spinal cord injury related - pathology.[29] It is available in a transdermal formulation for those who cannot tolerate oral usage.

ANTIHISTAMINE
Orphenadrine

The structure of orphenadrine is nearly identical to that of diphenhydramine with the addition of a methane group. It shares both antihistaminic and anticholinergic properties. It may be considered in patients with a history of bronchospasms/common allergies or Parkinson disease to reduce tremors and stiffness, respectively. Severe adverse effects include blurred vision, tachycardia, and urinary retention.[35]

PERIPHERALLY ACTING
Dantrolene

Dantrolene is the only known skeletal muscle relaxant that acts peripherally at the level of the striated muscle itself. It blocks the calcium release of the sarcoplasmic reticulum, which in turn, reduces extrafusal muscle fiber contractility and sensitivity.[23] It is known to exert the most influence on fast-twitch motor units.[29] It also exerts minor influence on smooth and cardiac muscle.

Skeletal Muscle Relaxants for Treatment of Acute and Chronic Low Back Pain

Skeletal muscle relaxants are frequently used in the treatment of acute and chronic back pain. According to Dillon and colleagues,[36] an estimated 2 million American adults reported muscle relaxant use. Of these, 85% of patients took muscle relaxants for treatment of low back pain or other muscle disorders. It is generally accepted to recommend a short course of skeletal muscle relaxants for treatment of acute low back pain. This is to take advantage of the properties of muscle relaxants that are deemed to reduce duration of discomfort while facilitating continued exertional activities to enhance recovery. Although most studies are historic, they have shown to be more effective than placebo for patients with acute low back pain with respect to short-term pain relief and functional outcomes.[37,38] The evidence for acute treatment for the aforementioned pharmacologic agents is less than a month.[39] Most clinical guidelines recommend use of skeletal muscle relaxants as either individual or adjuvant therapy. Often used alongside NSAIDs, there are studies that support the dual-therapy of cyclobenzaprine and NSAIDs.[23]

When deciding to institute a skeletal muscle relaxant for treatment of low back pain, one must take into account its chronicity. Dillon and colleagues[36] further elucidate upon the data available through National Health Nutrition Examination Survey (NHANES III), suggesting that the average length of use of muscle relaxants is 2.1 years,[37] and 44.5% of those who took muscle relaxants continued for more than a year.[38] More recent studies question the utility of skeletal muscle relaxants for management of chronic low back pain.[20,40] There are no current studies that demonstrate chronic low back pain relief or improvement in functional status to validate its long-term usage. However, this is a common practice among providers attributable to anecdotal success. Only a select group of patients with good ownership of self-management strategies with demonstration of functional improvement may benefit from chronic therapy. Providers should be mindful of the long-term adverse effects associated with skeletal muscle relaxants such as oversedation and CNS depression that are particularly seen in concomitant use of alcohol, anxiolytics, opioid, or other sedatives.[11] One hypothesis regarding patient-reported pain relief is that sedative effects and impaired cognition from use of skeletal muscle relaxants lead to increased reports of analgesia rather than direct effects of the medication.[41] In order to avoid inappropriate long-term use of muscle relaxants, patients suffering from chronic low back may benefit from an evaluation from a secondary provider and/or optimization of self-management strategies using an interdisciplinary pain program.

DISCLOSURE

The author has nothing to disclose.

REFERENCES

1. Elenbaas J. Centrally acting oral skeletal muscle relaxants. Am J Hosp Pharm 1980;37(10):1313–23.
2. Waldman HJ. Centrally acting skeletal muscle relaxants and associated drugs. J Pain Symptom Manage 1994;7:434–41.
3. Balano KB. Anti-inflammatory drugs and myorelaxants. Pharmacology and clinical use in musculoskeletal disease. Prim Care 1996;23(2):329–34.

4. Patel AT, Ogle AA. Diagnosis and management of acute low back pain. Am Fam Physician 2000;61:1779–86.
5. Honda M, Nishida T, Ono H, et al. Tricyclic analogs cyclobenzaprine, amitriptyline and cyproheptadine inhibit the spinal reflex transmission through 5-HT2 receptors. Eur J Pharmacol 2003;458(1–2):91–9.
6. Cyclobenzaprine ALZA Corp. 2001. Available at: https://www.accessdata.fda.gov/drugsatfda_docs/label/2003/017821s045lbl.pdf. Accessed January 29, 2020.
7. Carisoprodol MEDA Corp. 2007. Available at: https://www.accessdata.fda.gov/drugsatfda_docs/label/2009/011792s043lbl.pdf. Accessed January 29, 2020.
8. Johnson EW. The myth of skeletal muscle spasm. Am J Phys Med Rehabil 1989;68:1.
9. Rivner MH. The neurophysiology of myofascial pain syndrome. Curr Pain Headache Rep 2001;5(5):432–40.
10. Witenko C, Moorman-Li R, Motycka C, et al. Considerations for the appropriate use of skeletal muscle relaxants for the management of acute low back pain. P T 2014;39(6):427–35.
11. Chaghtai A, Argoff CE. Skeletal muscle relaxants and analgesic balms. Bonica's Management of Pain 2019;5:1352–8.
12. Fudin J, Raouf M. A review of skeletal muscle relaxants for pain management. Pract Pain Manage 2016;16(5):1–15.
13. Alvarex DJ, Rockwell PG. Trigger points: diagnosis and management. Am Fam Physician 2002;65(4):653–60.
14. Simons DG. Review of enigmatic MTrPs as a common cause of enigmatic musculoskeletal pain and dysfunction. J Electromyogr Kinesiol 2004;14(1):95–107.
15. Fathie K. A second look at a skeletal muscle relaxant: double-blind study of metaxalone. Curr Ther Res Clin Exp 1964;6:677–83.
16. Metaxalone king pharm. 2006. Available at: https://www.accessdata.fda.gov/drugsatfda_docs/label/2006/013217s046lbl.pdf. Accessed January 29, 2020.
17. Tisdale SA, Ervin DK. A controlled study of methocarbamol and acute painful musculoskeletal conditions. Curr Ther Res Clin Exp 1975;17(6):525–30.
18. Methocarbamol Baxter Corp. 2003. Available at: https://www.accessdata.fda.gov/drugsatfda_docs/label/2004/11790slr046_robaxin_lbl.pdf. Accessed January 29, 2020.
19. PDR Staff. Physicians' desk reference. 58th edition. New Jersey: PDR; 2004.
20. Reeves RR, Carter OS, Pinkofsky HB, et al. Carisoprodol: abuse potential and physician unawareness. J Addict Dis 1999;18(2):51–6.
21. Reeves RR, Carter OS, Pinkofsky HB, et al. Use of carisoprodol by substance abusers to modify the effects of illicit drugs. South Med J 1999;92(4):441.
22. Van Tulder MW, Touray T, Furlan AD, et al. muscle relaxants for nonspecific low back pain. Cochran Database Syst Rev 2003;(2):CD004252.
23. Flexeril [package insert]. Fort Washington (PA): McNeil Consumer and Specialty Pharmaceuticals; 2003.
24. Borenstein DG, Korn S. Efficacy of low-dose regimen of cyclobenzaprine hydrochloride and acute skeletal muscle spasm: results of 2 placebo-controlled trials. Clin Ther 2003;25(4):1056–73.
25. Browning R, Jackson JL, O'Malley PG. Cyclobenzaprine and back pain. A meta-analysis. Arch Intern Med 2001;161:1613–20.
26. Leite FM, Atallah AN, El Dib R, et al. Cyclobenzaprine for the treatment of myofascial pain in adults. Cochrane Database Syst Rev 2009;(3):CD006830.

27. Keegan MT, Brown DR, Rabinstein AA. Serotonin syndrome from the interaction of cyclobenzaprine with other serotonergic drugs. Anesth Analg 2006;103(6): 1466–8.

28. American Geriatrics Society Beers Criteria. 2015. Available at: https://www. guidelinecentral.com/summaries/american-geriatrics-society-2015-updated-beers-criteria-for-potentially-inappropriate-medication-use-in-older-adults/#section-420. Accessed January 29, 2020.

29. Cuccurullo SJ. Physical medicine and rehabilitation board review. 2nd edition. St Louis: Springer Publishing Company; 2009. p. 813–5.

30. Coward DM. Tizanidine: neuropharmacology and mechanism of action. Tizanidine: neuropharmacology and mechanism of action. Neurology 1994;44(11 supplemental 9):S6–10.

31. Smith HS, Barton AE. Tizanidine in the management of spasticity and musculoskeletal complaints in the palliative care population. Tizanidine in the management of spasticity and musculoskeletal complaints in the palliative care population. Am J Hosp Palliat Care 2000;17(1):50–8.

32. Malanga GA, Gwynn MW, Smith R, et al. Tizanidine is effective in the treatment of myofascial pain syndrome. Pain Physician 2002;5(4):422–32.

33. Berry H, Hutchinson DR. Tizanidine and ibuprofen in acute low back pain: results of a double-blind randomnized study in general practice. J Int Med Res 1988; 16(2):83–91.

34. Sirdalud Ternelin Asian Pacific Study Group. Efficacy and gastroprotective effects of tizanidine plus diclofenac versus placebo plus diclofenac in patients with painful muscle spasms. Curr Therap Res 1998;59(1):13–22.

35. Gold R. Orphenadrine citrate: sedative or muscle relaxant? Clin Ther 1978;1(6): 451–3.

36. Dillon C, Paulose-Ram R, Hirsch R, et al. Skeletal muscle relaxant use in the United States: date from the third National health and Nutrition examination surgery (NHANES III). Spine 2004;29(8):892–6.

37. Berry H, Hutchinson DR. A randomized placebo controlled study in general practice to evaluate the efficacy and safety of tizanidine acute low back pain. J Int Med Res 1988;16(2):75–82.

38. Barrata R. A double-blind study of cyclobenzaprine and placebo in the treatment of acute musculoskeletal condition of the low back. Curr Ther Res 1982;32(5): 646–52.

39. Chou R, Qaseem A, Snow V, et al. Clinical efficacy assessment subcommittee of the American College of Physicians, American Pain Society low back pain guidelines panel. Diagnosis and treatment of low back pain. Ann Intern Med 2007;147: 478–91.

40. Chou R, Peterson K, Helfand M. Comparative efficacy and safety of skeletal muscle relaxants for spasticity and musculoskeletal conditions: a systematic review. J Pain Symptom Manage 2004;28(2):140–75.

41. Hare BD, Lipman AG. Uses and misuses of medication in the treatment of chronic pain. Chronic pain, problems in Anesthesia. Philadelphia: JB Lippincott; 1990.

Pharmacologic Approach to Insomnia

Lina Fine, MD, MPhil

KEYWORDS

• Sleep • Insomnia • Hypnotic • Pain • Medication

KEY POINTS

- Sleep is closely involved in management of pain of symptoms, with a broad range of approaches available for management of insomnia.
- A majority of pharmacologic interventions focus on mediation at the γ-aminobutyric acid receptors.
- Novel pharmacologic agents aim at modulation of melatonin as well as orexin receptors.

RELATIONSHIP BETWEEN SLEEP AND PAIN

Sleep plays a vital role in management of pain symptomatology. Disruption in sleep patterns and architecture have been shown to worsen pain perception and lead to increased vulnerability to central sensitization, resulting in persistent, chronic pain.[1] The National Sleep Foundation in 2015 polled adults in order to understand sleep patterns and relationship of sleep to health, specifically, to pain perception and experience; 1031 responders were adults between ages of 18 and 92, with 52% of responders women; 65.5% percent were white, 11.6% were black, and 15.2% were Hispanic. Individuals who rated their health and quality of life more highly reported getting approximate 30 minutes more sleep on average in the preceding 7 days than those who rated their health or quality of life as poor or fair. Those respondents who reported experiencing pain the past 7 days slept less and had worse sleep quality than those who were pain-free. In the same population, pain also led to greater sleep debt, with 42 minutes reduction in total sleep in patients with chronic pain. People with chronic pain felt less in control of their sleep and worried more about effect of sleep on their health. Individuals with shorter sleep and greater sleep debt reported greater pain severity, especially in those with pain in 4 or more locations.

Those who reported chronic pain were significantly more likely to use sleep medication than those with no pain or those with acute pain.[2]

Swedish Sleep Medicine, 550 17 Avenue, Seattle, WA 98122, USA
E-mail address: lina.fine@swedish.org

Phys Med Rehabil Clin N Am 31 (2020) 255–264
https://doi.org/10.1016/j.pmr.2020.01.003
1047-9651/20/© 2020 Elsevier Inc. All rights reserved.

INSOMNIA DEFINITION, DIAGNOSIS, AND TREATMENT STANDARDS

Insomnia diagnosis encompasses the inability to initiate sleep, maintain sleep, or reach a state of restfulness and refreshment on awakening. It may be associated with daytime symptoms of fatigue, memory deficits, social/vocational/academic performance deficits, mood changes, daytime sleepiness, lack of motivation, vulnerability to accidents, and somatic symptoms. Current guidelines for management of insomnia set behavioral treatment of insomnia as the first-line approach to patients who may struggle with this sleep disorder.[3] Cognitive behavioral therapy (CBT) for insomnia (CBT-I) is the gold standard treatment of insomnia. CBT includes stimulus control therapy, relaxation therapy, or a combination of cognitive therapy, stimulus control therapy, and sleep restriction therapy with or without relaxation therapy. In acute insomnia (lasting <3 months) or in the setting of comorbid conditions, such as pain, however, pharmacologic therapy often is a major approach to treatment of insomnia and may be used in conjunction with CBT-I or as an alternative method of targeting this condition.

Insomnia assessment includes a thorough history of sleep complaints, medical and psychiatric history, and previous treatments, both pharmacologic and psychological, along with consideration of current medication management.[4] The 2016 American College of Physicians clinical practice guideline for insomnia recommended CBT-I as the initial intervention based on moderate-quality evidence, followed by reassessment for use of pharmacotherapy in patients who did not respond to behavioral therapy anchored in shared decision making.[5]

BENZODIAZEPINE RECEPTOR AGONISTS

Sleeping aids have been ubiquitous through the ages. In the nineteenth century, bromide salts, herbal supplements, opioid formulations, and alcohol were the treatments of choice. Barbiturates were added to the fray in the twentieth century but fell out of favor due to risks of lethal overdose and side effects. Chlordiazepoxide was the first benzodiazepine (BZD), introduced in 1963, followed by diazepam and then flurazepam in 1970. Flurazepam was the first BZD approved by Food and Drug Administration (FDA) as a sleeping aid. In 1992, non-BZD, γ-aminobutyric acid (GABA) receptor agonist zolpidem was approved. This non-BZD hypnotic remains the most widely prescribed hypnotic medication.[6]

BZD receptor agonists (BzRAs)include BZDs, such as triazolam and temazepam, and non-BZDs, known as Z-drugs, including zolpidem, eszopiclone, and zaleplon. Zolpidem is the most common prescribed hypnotic in this category. Both of these classes of drugs have a common mechanism of action that involves binding to BZD α-receptors of the GABA type A receptor complex. Binding to the receptor results in opening the chloride ion channel and facilitation of the inhibitory action of GABA, which is a widely distributed, inhibitory neurotransmitter in the central nervous system. BzRAs act allosterically, meaning that GABA also must be present on the receptor complex for BzRAs to have their inhibitory effects, which in part explains their wide therapeutic index.[7] In patients ages 18 years to 64 years, these hypnotics may be chosen as a short-term approach to management of insomnia. Although subjective improvement may be reported with these agents, odds of insomnia persistence despite BzRA use have been noted to be 2 times higher in patients with comorbid pain condition than in general population.[8]

Zolpidem and zaleplon have been reported to cause parasomnia-like episodes, including sleep eating, sleepwalking, and sleep driving. Coadministration with alcohol and administration at higher doses may lead to a higher risk of developing somnambulism (sleepwalking) and similar behaviors.[9–12] Used in conjunction with opioids, BzRAs may put patients at risk for sleep-disordered breathing, and screening for sleep apnea is advisable in these individuals.[13] BZD use in older individuals has been associated with higher risk of Alzheimer dementia (>65 years of age) in those using it on regular basis for 3 months or longer[14] (**Table 1**).

A shift away from BZD and non-BZD hypnotics occurred in the 1990s, when off-label use of sedating antidepressants, such as trazodone, significantly reduced prescription of hypnotics, with valid concerns for side effects and dependency risks of hypnotics.[15] There are few data of high quality to support use of sedating antidepressants, but these agents remain relevant in the arsenal of available sleep pharmacology.

SEDATIVE ANTIDEPRESSANTS
Trazodone—Heterocyclic Antidepressant

Trazodone is an antidepressant commonly used for sleep-onset insomnia and sleep-maintenance insomnia, at doses of 50 mg to 150 mg. The sedative effect of trazodone has been postulated to be mediated via α-adrenergic and mild histamine H_1 blocking actions. Despite paucity of data and absence of meta-analysis of this medication, it often is perceived as a safer choice and commonly used by clinicians.[16] This heterocyclic antidepressant has not been studied specifically in older patients. Trazodone

Table 1
Summary of benzodiazepine receptor agonists by indication

Name/Dose	Class	Sleep-Onset Insomnia	Sleep-Maintenance Insomnia
Temazepam/15 mg	BZD	37-min sleep latency reduction compared with placebo	99-min longer total sleep time compared with placebo; small improvement in sleep quality
Triazolam/0.25 mg	BZD	9-min sleep latency reduction compared with placebo	Not recommended
Zolpidem/10 mg*	non-BZD	5-12–min sleep latency reduction, compared with placebo	Total sleep time 29 min longer, wake after sleep onset: mean reduction was 25 min greater compared with placebo
Zaleplon/10 mg	non-BZD	10-min sleep latency reduction compared with placebo	Not recommended
Eszopiclone/2 mg or 3 mg	non-BZD	14-min sleep latency reduction compared with placebo	Total sleep time improvement 28–57 min longer, wake after sleep onset: mean reduction 10–14 min greater compared with placebo

*Note: FDA recommended dose for women is 5 mg
Data from Sateia MJ, Buysse DJ, Krystal AD, et al. Clinical Practice Guideline for the Pharmacologic Treatment of Chronic Insomnia in Adults: An American Academy of Sleep Medicine Clinical Practice Guideline. *J Clin Sleep Med*. 2017;13(2):307-349.

should be considered with caution in patients who may be already on 1 or more anti-depressants with mediating effect at serotonin receptors in order to minimize the risk of serotonin syndrome. Serotonin syndrome is a reaction to a combination of medications as a result of excessive activation of the postsynaptic serotonin receptors. Patients usually present with altered mental status (agitation, confusion, and hallucinations), autonomic instability (diaphoresis, shivering, and diarrhea) and neuro-muscular irritability (clonus, tremors, and fasciculations), with severity of symptoms varying from mild to life threatening. Although possible with overdose of a single sero-tonergic agent, it is most common in the interactions of 2 or more drugs acting at the serotonin receptors. The Hunter criteria for serotonin syndrome require 1 the following signs in a patient on at least 1 serotonergic agent: spontaneous clonus, inducible clonus plus agitation or diaphoresis, ocular clonus plus agitation or diaphoresis, and inducible clonus or ocular clonus plus hypertonia and hyperthermia.[17]

Doxepin—Tricyclic Antidepressant

Doxepin is a tricyclic antidepressant—a subcategory of heterocyclic antidepres-sants—that has been shown to be most effective in sleep-maintenance, insomnia at doses of 3 mg and 6 mg.[18] It has FDA-approved indications for insomnia. Headache and somnolence limited the use of this sedative in clinical trials. Other tricyclics, such as amitriptyline, have been used off-label to improve sleep but no quality data exist to support recommendation for systematic use of tricyclics, other than doxepin, for insomnia. Tricyclic antidepressants carry a risk of postural hypotension and slight pro-longation of QT interval that carries a risk in arrhythmia, especially in patients with car-diovascular disease.

Selective Serotonin Reuptake Inhibitors

Serotonin is involved in sleep-wake regulation, including transitions between specific sleep stages and the termination of rapid-eye-movement sleep. Drugs, such as selec-tive serotonin reuptake inhibitors (SSRIs), that modulate serotonin activity can lead to varied and significant effects on sleep. Fluoxetine, for example, can have sedating as well activating effects.[19] Placebo-controlled trial of paroxetine versus placebo, at dos-ages of 10 mg and 20 mg, showed increase in sleep latency and no difference in sleep efficacy[20] Given the diversity of SSRI effects on sleep, this class of medication should be considered with caution in individuals with insomnia.

Mirtazapine—Tetracyclic Antidepressant

Mirtazapine is a tetracyclic antidepressant with sleep promoting effects at lower doses. Mirtazapine may lead to statistically significant improvement in sleep effi-ciency, total sleep time, and sleep quality. The mechanism of action of mirtazapine is unique. It seems to exert its therapeutic effect via an overall increase in serotonin, norepinephrine, and dopamine levels, although not via the traditional blockade of re-uptake transporters.[21] Mirtazapine has its highest affinity for histaminergic H_1 recep-tors and serotonergic serotonin type 2A receptors. Blockade of H_1 provides sedating and anxiolytic properties, whereas blockade of serotonin type 2A receptors provides increased dopaminergic activity. At lower doses, histaminergic affinity leads to seda-tion whereas at higher doses, as more alpha$_2$ receptors become blocked and provide more of an activating effect through dopaminergic and noradrenergic signaling, the medication becomes more activating. Weak inverse relationship between mirtazapine concentration in plasma and sedation as well as increased sleep duration at low plasma concentration has been described.[22]

MELATONIN AGONIST: RAMELTEON

Ramelteon is a melatonin agonist that has been shown to provide improvement in sleep latency.[23] Melatonin is a neuropeptide produced by pineal gland in response to dim light and its production is regulated by circadian rhythms. This drug acts at the melatonin 1 (MT1) and melatonin 2 (MT2) receptors to promote sleep through effect on circadian rhythms. MT1 binding inhibits circadian-mediated wake-promoting activity. MT2 receptors are involved in timing of sleep. In contrast to other sleeping aids, ramelteon is not active at any central nervous system receptors commonly associated with sedation (GABA, dopamine, opiate, and serotonin). Perhaps due to this unique mechanism of action, ramelteon has demonstrated a low potential for abuse in clinical trials and may be valuable in patients who are at risk for substance abuse. It is the only insomnia therapeutic that is not classified as a scheduled drug by the US Drug Enforcement Administration. Meta-analytic data on adverse effects showed a relatively low frequency of adverse effects overall, none of which was significantly different than placebo, including in older population.[24]

OREXIN RECEPTOR ANTAGONISTS

The most novel entrants in the arena of the pharmacologic treatment of insomnia are orexin receptor agonists. Orexin is a neuropeptide produced by a group of neurons in lateral hypothalamus. Orexin plays an essential role in stabilizing wakefulness by acting on serotonin, histamine, acetylcholine, and dopamine.[25] Damage to this population of neurons may result in abrupt, often overwhelming, sleepiness. Narcolepsy is the condition in which orexin concentration is drastically reduced. The 2 new medications—suvorexant and lemborexant—target orexin receptors by blocking wake-promoting orexin.

Suvorexant

Suvorexant was the first dual orexin-A and orexin-B receptor antagonist to be approved by FDA and has demonstrated efficacy at decreasing both time to sleep onset and increasing total sleep time compared with placebo.[26] Objective reports of wake after sleep onset on polysomnogram showed clinically significant reduction at both 10 mg and 20 mg dosages, suggesting that suvorexant may improve sleep onset with effect more significant at higher dosages. There was no evidence of daytime residual or withdrawal symptoms.[27]

Lemborexant

Lemborexant is the most recent sleeping aid, approved by FDA at the end of 2019, for treatment of insomnia. Lemborexant is a competitive antagonist at orexin-A and orexin-B receptors that are involved in suppression of wake drive. According to phase III multicenter, randomized, double-blind, placebo-controlled, active comparator, parallel-group study of the efficacy and safety, lemborexant performed better than placebo for sleep-onset insomnia and sleep-maintenance insomnia.[28] It was tested specifically in subjects over 65 years of age and shown to have no statistically significant detriment in memory or driving ability the next day.[29]

ANTIEPILEPTIC DRUGS

Antiepileptic medications affect sleep architecture and influence the ability to fall and stay asleep. Gabapentin and tiagabine have been studied specifically in insomnia. Gabapentin has been studied in an open-label study and was found to enhance slow wave sleep in patients with primary insomnia. It also was found to improve sleep quality by elevating sleep efficiency and decreasing spontaneous arousals.[30] Tiagabine has been studied in primary insomnia and shown to have some limited efficacy in management of insomnia and was found to increase slow wave sleep.[31] Many other antiepileptic agents may have sedative properties but have not been studied in management of insomnia.

OTHER COMMONLY USED SLEEPING AIDS

Although not approved by FDA, multiple dietary supplements as well as medications with sedative effects have been tried for management of sleep-onset insomnia and sleep-maintenance insomnia. Over-the-counter supplements that have been tested and antiepileptic agents with evidence in management of insomnia have been included. Quetiapine has been used in clinical management of sleep difficulties in the context of anxiety and has been included in the context of anxiety management data.

OVER-THE-COUNTER AGENTS
Melatonin

Melatonin is available as a dietary supplement that is not regulated by FDA. Melatonin is a chronobiotic rather than hypnotic and is most effective in patients with circadian rhythm disorders, such as delayed sleep phase (night owls). Individuals with endogenous melatonin rhythm that is delayed to later time in the night compared with desired or required bedtime may benefit from low-dose (1 mg) melatonin at least 1 hour prior to bedtime. Administration of melatonin may advance sleep phase (move it to an earlier time) and improve sleep quality in the first tertile of sleep.[32]

Melatonin is the fourth most popular natural product taken by US adults (after fish oil/omega 3-fatty acids, glucosamine/chondroitin, and probiotics).[33] Lack of governmental oversight may lead to significant variability in the quality of melatonin and its dosing. Actual melatonin content (and presence of contaminants) in 31 melatonin supplements purchased from groceries and pharmacies in 1 city in Canada (before countrywide over-the-counter use of it in Canada was banned) found melatonin content to vary from −83% to +478% of labeled melatonin and 70% had melatonin concentration less than or equal to 10% of what was claimed. In addition, the content of melatonin between lots of the same product varied by as much as 465%.[34]

Diphenhydramine

Randomized clinical trials of diphenhydramine—a commonly used antihistamine—found that patient-reported sleep latency versus placebo fell below the level of clinically significant improvement.[35] Polysomnography-determined sleep latency and total sleep time showed outcomes, which also fell below clinical significance thresholds.[36] First-generation antihistamines, such as diphenhydramine, are associated with increased risk of dementia in older individuals (>65 years old) and, therefore, should be avoided.[37]

L-Tryptophan

L-tryptophan (ie, tryptophan) is 1 of 8 essential amino acids (ie, amino acids that cannot be synthesized in the human body and must be supplied by the diet) and is a precursor in serotonin synthesis.[38] L-tryptophan, based on patient-reported data, showed a modest decline in total sleep time, which was not clinically significant. Sleep quality was reported mildly, although not statistically significantly, increased.[39] On the basis of these findings, L-tryptophan is not recommended as a sleeping aid.

ATYPICAL ANTIPSYCHOTIS: QUETIAPINE

In patients with mental illness comorbidity, quetiapine, an atypical antipsychotic, at times is used due to its sedating effect. Atypical antipsychotics, however, are associated with increased risk of death in dementia-related psychosis in elderly patients.[40]

Alongside this risk, neuroleptic malignant syndrome should be considered due to its D_2 receptor blockage. The sedative effect of quetiapine comes from its strong antagonism at histamine (H_1) receptor. H_1 antagonism also is responsible for the side effect of weight gain of this medication.[41] Quetiapine may be helpful for management of generalized anxiety disorder that often coexists with insomnia and can precipitate insomnia. Three randomized control trials have shown the efficacy of treatment in monotherapeutic treatment over placebo. There is no FDA approval for use of quetiapine in anxiety, however, and further research is necessary to advocate for this indication.[42] Quetiapine is the least likely of atypical antipsychotics to cause extrapyramidal symptoms but it carries the risk of neuroleptic malignant syndrome and increased risk for suicidal ideation in patients with major depressive disorder.[43]

NONPHARMACOLOGIC APPROACH TO INSOMNIA

CBT-I is the primary recommended approach to management of insomnia because this treatment modality is more sustainable and carries a much lower risk for side effects than pharmacological approach. CBT-I leads to improvement in sleep-onset latency, time spent awake after sleep onset, sleep efficiency, and sleep quality as well as pain interference with daily functioning.[44] CBT-I includes

1. General education about the physiology of sleep, role of daylight and blue light, importance of a regular sleep-wake cycle, timing of caffeine intake, and alcohol intake
2. Bedtime restriction therapy that includes limiting the amount of time spent in bed to be equivalent to the average sleep time over 1 week and then increasing the sleep duration (or time in bed) gradually over several weeks. Wake-up time usually is kept steady in an attempt to also try to synchronize circadian rhythm.
3. Stimulus control is the use of classical conditioning to restrict the bedroom, especially the bed, to only sleep and intimacy, in order to associate the bedroom with sleepiness.
4. Sleep hygiene includes promoting sleep-inducing behaviors, including avoidance of caffeine, and timing of exercise.
5. Relaxation training and stress management involve guided visual imagery and breathing exercises that equip patients with tools to be used at night.
6. Sleep-focused cognitive therapy involves identifying maladaptive sleep-related beliefs and reframing them.[45]

SUMMARY

When considering a medication for sleep-related difficulty in adults with comorbid pain symptoms, it is helpful first to hone in on the exact nature of the complaint, specifically whether the patient reports sleep-onset difficulty at the initiation of sleep or sleep-maintenance insomnia with inability to resume sleep once awakened. The second consideration in this decision-making process is the choice of the class of medication to be chosen and its interaction with the patient's current pharmacologic regimen.

Third, the patient's age has become an important concern due to significant effect of several classes of drugs on patients who are over 65 years of age. BZDs and first-generation antihistamines, such as diphenhydramine—common sleeping aids—have been implicated in cognitive impairment in older individuals. The American Geriatric Society Beers Criteria advise that BZDs be avoided in treatment of insomnia in older patients due to risk of cognitive impairment, falls, and motor vehicle accidents.[46] The criteria also advise that BzRAs, such as zolpidem, be limited to shorter-term use of fewer than 90 days. Novel approaches, including orexin receptor agonists, may be safer and more promising pharmacologic approaches. Pharmacologic interventions, when used cautiously for a limited period of time and in complement with behavioral and cognitive approaches, can serve to improve sleep quality and significantly help in management of pain.

DISCLOSURE

The author has nothing to disclose.

REFERENCES

1. Smith MT, Edwards RR, McCann UD, et al. The effects of sleep deprivation on pain inhibition and spontaneous pain in women. Sleep 2007;30(4):494–505.
2. National Sleep Foundation. The 2015 Sleep in America poll. Available at: http://www.sleepfoundation.org.
3. Schutte-Rodin SL, Broch L, Buysee D, et al. Clinical guideline for the evaluation and management of chronic insomnia in adults. J Clin Sleep Med 2008;4(5):487–504.
4. Chesson A, Hartse K, Anderson WM, et al. Practice parameters for the evaluation of chronic insomnia. An American Academy of Sleep Medicine report. Standards of Practice Committee of the American Academy of Sleep Medicine. Sleep 2000;23(2):237–41. Available at: http://www.ncbi.nlm.nih.gov/pubmed/10737341. Accessed January 19, 2020.
5. Qaseem A, Kansagara D, Forciea MA, et al. Management of chronic insomnia disorder in adults: A clinical practice guideline from the American college of physicians. Ann Intern Med 2016;165(2):125–33.
6. Bertisch SM, Herzig SJ, Winkelman JW, et al. National use of prescription medications for insomnia: NHANES 1999-2010. Sleep 2014;37(2):343–9.
7. Roehrs T, Roth T. Insomnia pharmacotherapy. Neurotherapeutics 2012;9(4):728–38.
8. Pillai V, Roth T, Roehrs T, et al. Effectiveness of benzodiazepine receptor agonists in the treatment of insomnia: an examination of response and remission rates. Sleep 2017;40(2). https://doi.org/10.1093/sleep/zsw044.
9. Liskow B, Pikalov A. Zaleplon overdose associated with sleepwalking and complex behavior. J Am Acad Child Adolesc Psychiatry 2004;43(8):927–8.
10. Menkes DB. Triazolam-induced nocturnal bingeing with amnesia. Aust N Z J Psychiatry 1992;26(2):320–1.
11. Morgenthaler TI, Silber MH. Amnestic sleep-related eating disorder associated with zolpidem. Sleep Med 2002;3(4):323–7.
12. Lange CL. Medication-associated somnambulism. J Am Acad Child Adolesc Psychiatry 2005;44(3):211–2.
13. Marshansky S, Mayer P, Rizzo D, et al. Sleep, chronic pain, and opioid risk for apnea. Prog Neuropsychopharmacol Biol Psychiatry 2018;87(Pt B):234–44.

14. De Gage SB, Moride Y, Ducruet T, et al. Benzodiazepine use and risk of Alz-heimer's disease: Case-control study. BMJ 2014;349. https://doi.org/10.1136/bmj.g5205.

15. Roehrs T, Roth T. "Hypnotic" prescription patterns in a large managed-care pop-ulation. Sleep Med 2004;5(5):463–6.

16. Walsh JK, Erman M, Erwin CW, et al. Subjective hypnotic efficacy of trazodone and zolpidem in DSMIII-R primary insomnia. Hum Psychopharmacol Clin Exp 1998;13(3):191–8.

17. Wang RZ, Vashistha V, Kaur S, et al. Serotonin syndrome: preventing, recog-nizing, and treating it. Cleve Clin J Med 2016;83(11):810–7.

18. Krystal AD, Lankford A, Durrence HH, et al. Efficacy and safety of doxepin 3 and 6 mg in a 35-day sleep laboratory trial in adults with chronic primary insomnia. Sleep 2011;34(10):1433–42.

19. Beasley CM, Sayler ME, Weiss AM, et al. Fluoxetine: activating and sedating ef-fects at multiple fixed doses. J Clin Psychopharmacol 1992;12(5):328–33. Avail-able at: http://www.ncbi.nlm.nih.gov/pubmed/1479050. Accessed January 19, 2020.

20. Reynolds CF, Buysse DJ, Miller MD, et al. Paroxetine treatment of primary insomnia in older adults. Am J Geriatr Psychiatry 2006;14(9):803–7.

21. Millan MJ, Gobert A, Rivet JM, et al. Mirtazapine enhances frontocortical dopami-nergic and corticolimbic adrenergic, but not serotonergic, transmission by blockade of alpha2-adrenergic and serotonin2C receptors: a comparison with citalopram. Eur J Neurosci 2000;12(3):1079–95.

22. Grasmäder K, Verwohlt PL, Kühn K-U, et al. Relationship between mirtazapine dose, plasma concentration, response, and side effects in clinical practice. Phar-macopsychiatry 2005;38(3):113–7.

23. Mayer G, Wang-Weigand S, Roth-Schechter B, et al. Efficacy and safety of 6-month nightly ramelteon administration in adults with chronic primary insomnia. Sleep 2009;32(3):351–60.

24. Roth T, Seiden D, Wang-Weigand S, et al. A 2-night, 3-period, crossover study of ramelteon's efficacy and safety in older adults with chronic insomnia. Curr Med Res Opin 2007;23(5):1005–14.

25. Sutcliffe JG, de Lecea L. The hypocretins: excitatory neuromodulatory peptides for multiple homeostatic systems, including sleep and feeding. J Neurosci Res 2000;62(2):161–8.

26. Herring WJ, Snyder E, Budd K, et al. Orexin receptor antagonism for treatment of insomnia: A randomized clinical trial of suvorexant. Neurology 2012;79(23):2265–74.

27. Herring WJ, Connor KM, Ivgy-May N, et al. Suvorexant in patients with insomnia: results from two 3-month randomized controlled clinical trials. Biol Psychiatry 2016;79(2):136–48.

28. Rosenberg R, Murphy P, Zammit G, et al. Comparison of lemborexant with pla-cebo and zolpidem tartrate extended release for the treatment of older adults with insomnia disorder. JAMA Netw Open 2019;2(12):e1918254.

29. Vermeeren A, Jongen S, Murphy P, et al. On-the-road driving performance the morning after bedtime administration of lemborexant in healthy adult and elderly volunteers. Sleep 2019;42(4). https://doi.org/10.1093/sleep/zsy260.

30. Lo H-S, Yang C-M, Lo HG, et al. Treatment effects of gabapentin for primary insomnia. Clin Neuropharmacol 2010;33(2):84–90.

31. Walsh JK, Perlis M, Rosenthal M, et al. Tiagabine increases slow-wave sleep in a dose-dependent fashion without affecting traditional efficacy measures in adults

with primary insomnia. J Clin Sleep Med 2006;2(1):35–41. Available at: http://www.ncbi.nlm.nih.gov/pubmed/17557435. Accessed January 19, 2020.

32. Sletten TL, Magee M, Murray JM, et al. Efficacy of melatonin with behavioural sleep-wake scheduling for delayed sleep-wake phase disorder: A double-blind, randomised clinical trial. PLoS Med 2018;15(6). https://doi.org/10.1371/journal.pmed.1002587.

33. Black LI, Clarke TC, Barnes PM, et al. Use of complementary health approaches among children aged 4-17 years in the United States: National Health Interview Survey, 2007-2012. Natl Health Stat Report 2015;(78):1–19. Available at: http://www.ncbi.nlm.nih.gov/pubmed/25671583. Accessed January 19, 2020.

34. Erland LAE, Saxena PK. Melatonin natural health products and supplements: presence of serotonin and significant variability of melatonin content. J Clin Sleep Med 2017;13(2):275–81.

35. Glass JR, Sproule BA, Herrmann N, et al. Effects of 2-week treatment with temazepam and diphenhydramine in elderly insomniacs: a randomized, placebo-controlled trial. J Clin Psychopharmacol 2008;28(2):182–8.

36. Morin CM, Koetter U, Bastien C, et al. Valerian-hops combination and diphenhydramine for treating insomnia: a randomized placebo-controlled clinical trial. Sleep 2005;28(11):1465–71.

37. Gray SL, Anderson ML, Dublin S, et al. Cumulative use of strong anticholinergics and incident dementia: A prospective cohort study. JAMA Intern Med 2015;175(3):401–7.

38. Wurtman RJ, Hefti F, Melamed E. Precursor control of neurotransmitter synthesis. Pharmacol Rev 1980;32(4):315–35. Available at: http://www.ncbi.nlm.nih.gov/pubmed/6115400. Accessed January 19, 2020.

39. Hudson C, Hudson SP, Hecht T, et al. Protein source tryptophan versus pharmaceutical grade tryptophan as an efficacious treatment for chronic insomnia. Nutr Neurosci 2005;8(2):121–7.

40. Maust DT, Kim HM, Seyfried LS, et al. Antipsychotics, other psychotropics, and the risk of death in patients with dementia. JAMA Psychiatry 2015;72(5):438.

41. Schatzberg AF, Nemeroff CB, American Psychiatric Association Publishing. The American Psychiatric Association Publishing Textbook of Psychopharmacology. Available at: https://www.appi.org/american_psychiatric_association_publishing_textbook_of_psychopharmacology_fifth_edition. Accessed January 19, 2020.

42. Maneeton N, Maneeton B, Woottiluk P, et al. Quetiapine monotherapy in acute treatment of generalized anxiety disorder: a systematic review and meta-analysis of randomized controlled trials. Drug Des Devel Ther 2016;10:259–76.

43. Solmi M, Murru A, Pacchiarotti I, et al. Safety, tolerability, and risks associated with first- and second-generation antipsychotics: a state-of-the-art clinical review. Ther Clin Risk Manag 2017;13:757–77.

44. Finan PH, Buenaver LF, Runko VT, et al. Cognitive-behavioral therapy for comorbid insomnia and chronic pain. Sleep Med Clin 2014;9(2):261–74.

45. Nijs J, Mairesse O, Neu D, et al. Sleep disturbances in chronic pain: Neurobiology, assessment, and treatment in physical therapist practice. Phys Ther 2018;98(5):325–35.

46. By the 2019 American Geriatrics Society Beers Criteria® Update Expert Panel. American Geriatrics Society 2019 updated AGS beers criteria® for potentially inappropriate medication use in older adults. J Am Geriatr Soc 2019;67(4):674–94.

Opioid Management
Initiating, Monitoring, and Tapering

W. Michael Hooten, MD

KEYWORDS

- Chronic pain • Opioid • Long-term opioid • Therapy

KEY POINTS

- A detailed medical and mental health evaluation before initiating long-term opioid therapy is needed to determine the patient's candidacy for long-term opioid therapy.
- The least potent drug prescribed at the lowest effective dose should be the general aim of treatment.
- The CAREFUL acronym is a pragmatic tool that is used in daily clinical practice to guide the assessment and documentation of many key components of clinical surveillance recommended in the CDC guidelines.
- Consensual tapering, defined as mutual agreement between the patient and clinician to taper opioids, is generally safe and effective. Nonconsensual tapering, defined as lack of patient consent or agreement to taper opioids, has been associated with a broad array of adverse effects including suicide.

INTRODUCTION

In recent years, numerous guidelines targeting the safe use of opioids for chronic pain have been published. The most influential guideline published to date is the Centers for Disease Control and Prevention (CDC) Guideline for Prescribing Opioids for Chronic Pain.[1] However, substantial challenges persist in the clinical application of best practice recommendations provided by the CDC and other guidelines.[2] Therefore, the purpose of this article is to describe a pragmatic approach to the clinical care of adults with chronic pain receiving long-term opioid therapy. This article is comprised of three sections. The first section focuses on key components of the clinical evaluation before initiating long-term opioid therapy. The second section highlights the importance of identifying individual patient characteristics that should be considered when initiating opioid therapy; and provides a simple acronym for organizing and documenting the clinical surveillance of long-term opioid therapy. The final section outlines several approaches to discontinuing opioid therapy including the potential risks and benefits of this aspect of patient care.

Department of Anesthesiology and Perioperative Medicine, Mayo Clinic, Charlton 1-145, 200 First Street SW, Rochester, MN 55905, USA
E-mail address: hooten.william@mayo.edu

Phys Med Rehabil Clin N Am 31 (2020) 265–277
https://doi.org/10.1016/j.pmr.2020.01.006
pmr.theclinics.com

This review is not intended to supplant previously published guidelines, specifically, the CDC guidelines. Rather, this review is intended to build on current knowledge to drive the clinical implementation of previously established best practice recommendations for the care of adults receiving long-term opioid therapy.

CLINICAL EVALUATION BEFORE INITIATING OPIOID THERAPY
Pain Pathways

A constellation of spinal cord and brain regions are activated by pain stimuli. This is important because receptors for endogenous opioids are located in the periphery, the dorsal root ganglion, the spinal cord, and the brain. A growing body of research suggests that pain stimuli are processed by a three-tiered neural network that encompasses the initial encoding of pain stimuli and extends to include the conscious modulation and memory formation of the pain experience (**Fig. 1**).[3,4] Peripheral nociceptors are activated by noxious stimuli. These stimuli are transmitted by primary afferents to the dorsal root ganglion and then on to the dorsal horn of the spinal cord. In the dorsal horn, the spinothalamic tract is activated and pain stimuli are transmitted to the posterior thalamus. Pain stimuli undergo further processing in the anterior cingulate cortex, insula, prefrontal cortex, and posterior parietal cortex. As a result, pain stimuli are consciously perceived, subjected to cognitive modulation, and transformed into somatic responses. In a related group of neural structures, pain perception is further modulated by the emotional context of the stimuli and individualized by psychological factors that influence memory formation. These cortical regions interact with descending spinal cord tracts to either inhibit or facilitate modulation of incoming pain stimuli.

Opioid Pharmacology

Opioids bind a 7-transmembrane G-protein coupled receptor in the central nervous system and results in hyperpolarization of the cell membrane, inhibition of adenylate cyclase, decreased intracellular cAMP, and reductions in the release of neurotransmitters associated with nociception.[5] Three receptors with distinct pharmacologic effects have been identified including the *mu-*, *delta*, and *kappa*-opioid receptor (**Table 1**).[6] Agonist activity at the mu-opioid receptor results in hyperpolarization of the membrane, inhibition of adenylate cyclase, and decreased intracellular cAMP. This cascade of intracellular reactions reduces the release of neurotransmitters (eg, substance P, γ-aminobutyric acid, dopamine, acetylcholine, and norepinephrine) that play key roles in nociception.

History and Physical Examination

Before initiating opioid therapy, a complete history and physical examination should be performed. One of the key aspects of the initial examination is to establish the primary pain diagnosis that is the indication for opioid therapy, which facilitates a targeted assessment of pain intensity. Clearly identifying the primary pain diagnosis also allows the clinician to fully optimize evidence-supported nonopioid pharmacotherapy and nonpharmacologic therapies before initiating opioids. Other important components of the initial history and physical examination include identification of co-morbid medical problems that could alter drug metabolism and potentially increase the risk of adverse effects. For example, baseline serologic measures of renal and hepatic function should be assessed in patients with known or suspected renal insufficiency or hepatic dysfunction. Similarly, individuals with pulmonary disease or sleep-disordered breathing should be carefully assessed to ensure the respiratory

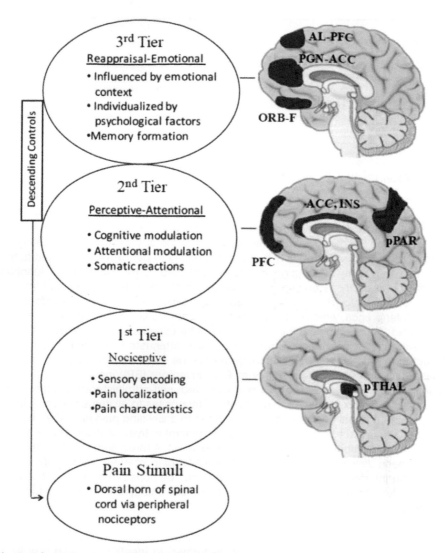

Fig. 1. Schematic representation of three-tiered pain matrix. ACC, anterior cingulate cortex; AL-PFC, anterolateral prefrontal cortex; INS, insula; ORB-F, orbitofrontal; PFC, prefrontal cortex; PGN, perigenual ACC; pPAR, posterior parietal cortex; pTHAL, posterior thalamus. (*From* Hooten WH. Chronic pain and mental health disorders: shared neural mechanisms, epidemiology, and treatment. Mayo Clinic Proceedings. 2016; 91(7):955-970; with permission.)

depressant effects of opioids do not worsen pulmonary function or sleep-related problems. Finally, use of concurrent medications should be carefully assessed to mitigate the risk of adverse drug-drug interactions. Because of the risk of accidental overdose associated with concurrent use of benzodiazepines and opioids,[7] use of benzodiazepines should be thoroughly assessed including review of prescription monitoring databases. Although the CDC guidelines clearly discourage coprescribing of opioids and benzodiazepines, prescribing patterns have only been modestly impacted since publication of the guidelines.[8] A urine toxicology screen should be considered if the current status of benzodiazepine use remains indeterminate.

Table 1 Opioid receptor class and effects	
Receptor Class	Effects
Mu	Analgesia, euphoria, addiction potential, confusion, dizziness nausea, respiratory depression, miosis, urinary retention, constipation, physical dependence
Delta	Analgesia, cardiovascular depression, constipation, respiratory depression
Kappa	Analgesia, dysphoria, hallucinations, delusions, sedation

Pain and Functional Assessment

An assessment of pain and functioning should be obtained before initiating opioid therapy. A functional assessment generally implies determining the capacity of an individual to perform physical activities. Critical domains of physical functioning that should be assessed before initiating opioid therapy include the capacity to perform routine activities of daily living, the capacity to perform work-related activities, and the ability to engage in leisure activities. Other domains of function include the capacity to engage in social and family activities. Functional impairments related to fixed anatomic or neurologic problems are further confounded by pain interference, which is defined as the extent to which pain limits engagement in activities. Although opioid therapy would not be expected to alter fixed anatomic or neurologic deficits, effective treatment should attenuate functional impairments attributed to pain interference. Although numerous questionnaires are available to assess pain and functioning, the Brief Pain Inventory (BPI) incorporates both of these clinical parameters. The BPI is a validated, self-administered questionnaire that takes less than 5 minutes to complete.[9] Responses to all items are completed using 10-point visual analog scales. In addition to assessing pain intensity, the BPI assesses the impact of pain interference on general activity, walking ability, work-related activities, social activities, and life enjoyment. A three-item short-form of the BPI has been developed. The PEG (Pain intensity; pain interference with life Enjoyment; pain interference with General activity) has demonstrated construct validity comparable with the BPI and it is used to detect changes in pain and function over time.[10]

Mental Health Evaluation

A mental health assessment should be performed to identify potential problems that increase the risk for problematic opioid use or opioid use disorder (OUD). Because of the paucity of mental health services in the ambulatory care setting, several key factors can be readily assessed by the nonmental health professional. For example, a mental health history should be obtained from the patient and the medical record should be carefully reviewed. Important aspects of this history include previous diagnosis of a psychiatric disorder, prior psychiatric hospitalization, prior admissions for alcohol or other substance detoxification, and previous suicide attempts. In addition, a review of current and previously prescribed psychotropic medications could also provide important information about prior episodes of psychiatric care.

When a psychiatric disorder is suspected in the absence of a past history of mental health care, several screening instruments are available to assess for depression, anxiety, and substance use disorders (**Table 2**).[3] Two brief screening questionnaires that are widely used in the primary care setting are the two-item Patient Health

Table 2
Sensitivities and specificities of screening questionnaire cutoff scores for depression, anxiety, and substance use disorders

	Cutoff Score	Sensitivity (%)	Specificity (%)
Depression			
Beck Depression Inventory	15	77	61
Hamilton Rating Scale for Depression	17	81	65
Center for Epidemiologic Studies Depression Scale	27	82	68
Patient Health Questionnaire Depression	10	79	60
Anxiety			
Hospital Anxiety and Depression Scale-Anxiety	8	88	81
Beck Anxiety Inventory	5.5	76	77
Patient Health Questionnaire Anxiety (Generalized Anxiety Disorder-7)	10	89	82
Substance use disorders			
Alcohol Use Identification Test	8	88	77
CAGE (alcohol)	2	71	90

Modified from Hooten WH. Chronic pain and mental health disorders: shared neural mechanisms, epidemiology, and treatment. Mayo Clinic Proceedings. 2016; 91(7):955-970; with permission.

Questionnaire[11] (PHQ-2), which is used to screen for depression, and the two-item Generalized Anxiety Disorder[12] (GAD-2) questionnaire. The PHQ-2 and the GAD-2 use the same lead question: "Over the past 2 weeks, how often have you been bothered by the following problems?" Responses to the following two questions are used to score the PHQ-2: "Little interest or pleasure in doing things" and "Feeling down, depressed or hopeless." Each question is scored from zero, indicating "not at all," to three, indicating "nearly every day." A score greater than or equal to three has a sensitivity and specificity of 83% and 90%, respectively, for major depressive disorder and a sensitivity and specificity of 62% and 95%, respectively, for any depressive disorder.[11] Similar to the PHQ-2, responses to the following two questions are used to score the GAD-2: "Feeling nervous, anxious or on edge" and "Not being able to stop or control worrying." The GAD-2 and the PHQ-2 use the same scoring scheme. A score greater than or equal to three has a sensitivity and specificity of 86% and 83%, respectively, for generalized anxiety disorder and a sensitivity and specificity of 65% and 88%, respectively, for any anxiety disorder.[12]

If clinically suspected, patients should also be screened for substance use disorders. Although numerous screening instruments are available (see **Table 2**), most only screen for a single substance. The Tobacco, Alcohol, Prescription Medication, and other Substance use (TAPS) tool screens for multiple substances and provides a substance-specific risk assessment for positive screen results.[13] The TAPS is supported by the National Institute on Drug Abuse, and clinician and patient versions are available online.[14] A score greater than or equal to one on the self-administered TAPS has a sensitivity and specificity of 77% for problem alcohol use, a sensitivity and specificity of 61% and 98% for problem opioid use, and a sensitivity and specificity of 82% and 75% for any substance use problem.[13] A urine toxicology screen should be considered if the substance use status is indeterminate or if relapse to substance use is clinically suspected.

Screening Tools to Predict Problematic Opioid Use

Screening for psychiatric disorders, including substance use disorders, that are associated with problematic opioid use should be distinguished from screening tools specifically designed to assess, or predict, the risk of developing opioid use–related problems. In general, the operating characteristics of these targeted screening tools are poor and this was acknowledged in the CDC guidelines[1(p29)]:

> Previous guidelines have recommended screening or risk assessment tools to identify patients at higher risk for misuse or abuse of opioids. However, the clinical evidence review found that currently available risk-stratification tools (e.g., Opioid Risk Tool, Screener and Opioid Assessment for Patients with Pain Version 1, SOAPP-R, and Brief Risk Interview) show insufficient accuracy for classification of patients as at low or high risk for abuse or misuse.

For example, the sensitivity and specificity of the Opioid Risk Tool for predicting development of opioid use–related problems is 25% and 85%, respectively.[15] Furthermore, the positive predictive value is 10% and the positive likelihood ratio is 1.5.[15] The operating characteristics of the Screener and Opioid Assessment for Patients with Pain Version 1 are similarly poor: sensitivity 59%, specificity 48%, positive predictive value 8%, and positive likelihood ratio 1.2.[16] Consistent with the content of the CDC guidelines, these type of measures should be used with caution.

Establishing Goals of Opioid Therapy

Before initiating a trial of opioid therapy, realistic expectations for pain relief, functional improvements, and potential adverse medication effects should be openly discussed including the risks of an accidental overdose, death, and development of OUD. This encounter should also include a discussion about the initial duration of therapy and plans to discontinue opioids if the goals of treatment are not met. Many ambulatory care clinics and health care delivery systems use opioid contracts, which are nonlegally binding agreements signed by the patient and clinician. In general, opioid contracts outline the responsibilities of the patient and clinician, and provide documentation that the goals, risks and benefits, and duration of therapy have been discussed. The potential benefits of opioid contracts in deterring aberrant drug-related behaviors has been brought into question by the results of a recently published systematic review.[17]

INITIATION AND SURVEILLANCE OF OPIOID THERAPY
Imitation of Opioid Therapy

The least potent drug prescribed at the lowest effective dose should be the general aim of treatment. Because the clinical problem is chronic pain and not acute pain, a patient's desire for prompt analgesia should be carefully assessed to avoid the risks associated with a rapid dose titration including respiratory depression. The initial dose should be prescribed when the patient does not have any scheduled activities because of the potential occurrence of an acute adverse effect (eg, nausea or sedation). Comorbid medical conditions should guide selection of the most appropriate medication and long-acting agents should be strictly avoided in opioid naive patients (Table 3). For tramadol and tapentadol, an initial dose of 50 mg followed by a second 50-mg dose 12 hours later is a reasonable regimen especially for adults greater than 65 years of age. Although any dose titration should be individualized, the dose of each drug could then be increased by 50 mg every 3 to 4 days. For hydrocodone and immediate release oxycodone, an initial dose of 5 mg followed by a second 5-mg dose

Table 3
Properties of commonly prescribed shorting-acting opioids

Opioid	Description	Morphine Equivalency	Half-Life	Metabolites	Safety Considerations
Hydrocodone	Oral, semisynthetic, 36% protein-bound	1:1	3–4 h	Norhydrocodone (CYP3A4) Hydromorphone (CYP2D6)	Mainly renal excretion
Hydromor-phone	Semisynthetic; multiple formulations available	1:5	2–3 h	H3G (direct conjugation)	High potency restricts use as first-line agent
Morphine	Derived from the poppy seed; multiple formulations available	Not applicable	2.5–4 h	M3G, M6G (direct conjugation) Normorphine (CYP3A4)	M6G more potent and longer acting than parent compound
Oxycodone	Oral, semisynthetic, 45% protein bound	1:1.1	3.2 h	Noroxycodone (CYP3A4) Noroxymorphone (CYP2D6, CYP3A4) Oxymorphone (CYP2D6)	Improved toxicity in patients with impaired renal or hepatic function
Tapentadol	Oral, synthetic, *mu*-receptor agonist and NE reuptake inhibition	4:1	4 h (IR)	Inactive metabolites via direct conjugation, CYP2C9, CYP2C19, CYP2D6	Weak muscarinic and 5-HT3 antagonist; no effect on cP450 enzymes
Tramadol	Oral, synthetic codeine analogue, 20% protein bound; *mu*-receptor agonist and NE reuptake inhibition	5:1	6.0–7.5 h	Single active metabolite M1, derived from O-methylation mediated by CYP2D6	Caution with impaired CYP2D6 activity

Abbreviations: 5HT3, serotonin; H3G, hydromorphine-3-glucuronide; M3G, morphine-3-glucuronide; M6G, morphine-6-glucuronide; NE, norepinephrine.

12 hours later is a safe initial dosing regimen that is not expected to have any significant respiratory depressant effects. The dose of each drug could then be increased by 5 mg every 3 to 4 days. A follow-up evaluation should be scheduled 10 to 14 days following initiation of therapy or sooner if clinically indicated.

Clinical Surveillance During Long-Term Opioid Therapy

Key components of the CDC guidelines center around best practices for maintaining long-term opioid therapy. Maintenance of best practices provides the framework for identifying potential complications including opioid misuse and OUD. Application of the CDC guidelines in daily clinical practice is often difficult to operationalize but the CAREFUL acronym (**Box 1**) provides a summary of many key components of clinical surveillance recommended in the CDC guidelines.[18]

Although use of opioid contracts (C in CAREFUL acronym) has been previously discussed, it should be emphasized that these agreements specify shared responsibilities between the patient and clinician. This is important because the responsibilities of clinicians are often overlooked.

Despite assessing for addiction (A in CAREFUL) before initiation of opioid therapy, all patients should be assessed during the course of therapy to identify early signs and symptoms of opioid misuse or OUD. One important surveillance method that provides objective data about controlled substance use is prescription drug monitoring programs (R_x in CAREFUL), which are now available in all 50 states and the District of Columbia. These online databases of dispensed controlled substances should be checked whenever an opioid prescription renewal is issued.

The opioid dose should be regularly assessed to ensure the effective (E in CAREFUL) lowest dose is being prescribed. Although dosing regimens are typically individualized, doses greater than 50 morphine milligram equivalents have been associated with accidental overdoses. An important determinant of the effective lowest dose is functionality (F in CAREFUL) including pain intensity. The three-item PEG questionnaire is sensitive to changes in pain and pain interference over time.

Similar to prescription drug monitoring programs, urine drug screens (U in CAREFUL) provide an objective measure of medication compliance including the use of other controlled and illicit substances. Aberrant urine drug screen results during the course of therapy could help identify an emerging substance use problem including OUD. Although the CDC guidelines recommend at least one urine drug screen annually, obtaining a screen every 3 to 4 months could enhance early detection of an evolving problem.

Finally, longitudinal follow-up (L in CAREFUL) is the cornerstone of clinical surveillance because all other surveillance interventions are dependent on face-to-face encounters with the patient. The frequency of follow-up was not specified in the CDC guidelines, but regularly scheduled appointments every 1 to 3 months should provide ample opportunities to document an accurate account of the patient's clinical course. Thus, the CAREFUL acronym is a pragmatic tool that is used in daily clinical practice to guide the assessment and documentation of many key components of clinical surveillance recommended in the CDC guidelines.

Monitoring Endocrine Function During Opioid Therapy

Opioid use is associated with a broad range of endocrinopathies. Opioids inhibit the entire hypothalamic-pituitary-gonadal axis by binding to opioid receptors in the

---

Box 1
The CAREFUL acronym for the clinical surveillance of long-term opioid therapy

C	Contract for opioid use
A	Addiction risk
R	R_x monitoring programs
E	Effective lowest dose
F	Functionality
U	Urine drug screen
L	Longitudinal follow-up

From Hooten WH. CAREFUL: a practical guide for improving the clinical surveillance of long-term opioid therapy. Mayo Clinic Proceedings. 2018; 93(8):1149; with permission.

hypothalamus, which decreases the secretion of gonadotropin-releasing hormone.[19] Commonly occurring signs of hypogonadism include diminished libido and sexual functioning, infertility, fatigue, and loss of muscle mass and strength. Opioids also inhibit the hypothalamic-pituitary-adrenal axis by directly suppressing adrenal function, and by suppressing the production of corticotropin-releasing hormone and adrenocorticotropic hormone.[19,20] Commonly occurring signs of adrenal insufficiency include fatigue, weight loss, dizziness, and diffuse myalgia. Many of the signs and symptoms of hypogonadism and adrenal insufficiency overlap with symptoms that are frequently associated with chronic pain. Thus, serologic monitoring for hypogonadism[19] (eg, total and free testosterone in men, estradiol in women) and adrenal insufficiency[20] (eg, cortisol, corticotropin, and corticotropin stimulation test) should be considered if clinically indicated. However, because of the diurnal variation in hormone levels and complexities associated with accurately interpreting the test results, referral to an endocrinologist may be warranted.

TERMINATION OF LONG-TERM OPIOID THERAPY
Indications for Opioid Tapering

Widely accepted indications for tapering long-term opioid therapy have not been fully established, aside from a patient's request to discontinue therapy. However, the indications for tapering are loosely grouped into three categories.[21,22] The first category is comprised of clinical factors indicating that the goals of treatment were not met. For example, inadequate pain reduction in the context of diminishing analgesia; lack of functional improvement; and progression of pain interference in physical, emotional, and social functioning. The second category is comprised of changes in the patient's medical status that increases the risk of potential opioid-related adverse effects. For example, deterioration of renal or hepatic function may necessitate dose reductions or tapering to reduce the risk of toxicity because of high serum drug levels. Similarly, the diagnosis of a central nervous system disease (ie, Parkinson disease, stroke, Alzheimer disease) may necessitate dose reductions or tapering to reduce the risk of delirium or other adverse neurologic effects. The third category is comprised of signs and symptoms indicative of opioid misuse, OUD, or identification of drug diversion. A pocket guide for opioid tapering is available online from the CDC.[22]

Risks of Tapering Long-Term Opioids

A chief determinant of risk in long-term opioid tapering is patient consent. Consensual tapering, defined as mutual agreement between the patient and clinician to taper opioids, is generally safe and effective. Nonconsensual tapering, defined as lack of patient consent or agreement to taper opioids, has been associated with a broad array of adverse effects including failure to complete the taper, termination of care, overdose, suicidal ideation, worsening depression and anxiety, and increased use of hospital and emergency department services.[23–25] However, patient-related factors (eg, OUD, opioid misuse) that precipitated opioid discontinuation may play an independent causal role in the harms associated with tapering.

Other factors associated with unsuccessful tapering include fear of acute opioid withdrawal and increased pain following opioid discontinuation. Although acute opioid withdrawal in ambulatory patients is a nonlethal withdrawal state, signs and symptoms of withdrawal should be carefully followed to reduce the risk of patient dropout during the taper. Commonly encountered physical symptoms include restlessness, sleep disruption, diaphoresis, rhinorrhea, yawning, nausea, loose stool, pupillary dilation, piloerection, and elevated blood pressure and heart rate. Affective distress, characterized by acute dysphoria and anxiety, are often observed. Finally, because of activation of descending pain facilitatory tracts during opioid tapering, patients may report diffuse arthralgia and myalgia with or without acute exacerbation of baseline pain symptoms.

Opioid Taper Schedules and Treatment of Acute Withdrawal

Evidence-supported opioid tapering schedules do not currently exist. However, several approaches based on percent dose reduction are used in the outpatient setting. In general, these approaches suggest reducing the baseline dose by 5% to 10% followed by similar dose reductions based, in part, on the indication for opioid tapering.[22,26,27] When the indication for tapering requires rapid dose reduction (ie, acute change in the patient's medical status, patient safety at risk because of unsafe opioid use), dose reductions of 5% to 10% may occur every 2 to 3 days to every week. Rapid tapering intended to protect patient safety is generally nonconsensual and occurs in the context of opioid misuse, OUD, or following an accidental overdose. If the indication for tapering is consensual, dose reductions of 5% to 10% may occur every week, biweekly or every month. In these clinical scenarios where the duration of the taper is not time sensitive, the frequency of dose reductions should be carefully discussed and planned with the patient. This enhances patient trust, reduces anticipatory anxiety about the taper, and provides adequate opportunities to provide other nonopioid-based treatments for pain as clinically indicated.

In the context of consensual tapering, slow dose reductions should mitigate the risk of acute opioid withdrawal. In these clinical scenarios, acute opioid withdrawal is easily treated by (1) temporarily providing additional small doses of opioid until the symptoms abate; (2) temporarily increasing the dose; or (3) increasing the frequency of further dose reductions. In the context of a rapid taper, several adjunct medications are available. α_2-Agonists reduce symptoms of acute opioid withdrawal by, in part, reducing the activity of the sympathetic nervous system.[28] Oral clonidine at doses of 0.05 mg to 0.1 mg every 6 to 12 hours is widely used but the drug should be carefully titrated because of adverse effects including hypotension and bradycardia. These adverse effects may be accentuated in the context of acute withdrawal, which can be associated with hypovolemia caused by the gastrointestinal effects of the withdrawal state. Another α_2-agonist is lofexidine, which is widely used in Europe and was recently approved by the Food and Drug Administration for acute opioid withdrawal.[29] Lofexidine is typically dosed at 0.54 mg every 6 hours. Similar to clonidine, commonly occurring adverse effects include hypotension, bradycardia, and dizziness. Other medications of varying mechanisms have been used to treat acute withdrawal including gabapentin[30]; trazodone[31]; low-dose naltrexone combined with clonidine[32]; and loperamide, but use of this drug at higher doses can cause arrhythmias.[33]

In addition to the pharmacologic management of acute opioid withdrawal, nonpharmacologic interventions should be considered including supportive therapy, cognitive behavioral therapy, use of stress-reduction techniques, meditation, pain and withdrawal-related psychoeducation, and graded exercise.[34]

Clinical Outcomes of Opioid Tapering

Recently, interest in the long-term outcomes of opioid tapering has grown. In a systematic review that involved 67 studies focusing on opioid reduction and discontinuation, significant improvements in pain severity (eight of eight studies), function (five of five studies), and quality of life (three of three studies) were observed.[35] The quality of evidence supporting these clinical observations was assessed as fair. In a separate systematic review, it was hypothesized that pain improves or does not change following opioid tapering.[36]

This review included 20 studies that involved a total of 2109 patients. Study inclusion criteria included reporting pretaper and posttaper pain scores and exclusion criteria included use of an opioid substitution. Sixteen studies reported improved pain posttapering, three studies reported that pain was unchanged posttapering, and a single study reported that pain was unchanged or improved in 97% of patients and worse in 3% of patients. In summary, these systematic reviews suggest that opioid tapering is associated with longer-term improvements in pain and functionality.

SUMMARY

As the national crisis of opioid-related morbidity and mortality persists, approaches to increase the uptake of best practice recommendations are needed. The pragmatic approaches set forth in this review could be one small step toward operationalizing these recommendations for implementation in daily clinical practice. However, a pressing need exists for ongoing research to further clarify the optimal role that long-term opioid therapy has in the treatment of chronic pain.

ACKNOWLEDGMENTS

The author would like to acknowledge Christine Hunt, DO for assisting with table development.

DISCLOSURE

Dr W.M. Hooten receives funding from the NIH and he has an unrestricted grant from US WorldMeds for an open label study of the effects of lofexidine on acute opioid withdrawal.

REFERENCES

1. Dowell D, Haegerich TM, Chou R. CDC guideline for prescribing opioids for chronic pain—United States, 2016. MMWR Recomm Rep 2016;65:1–49.
2. Kroenke K, Alford DP, Argoff C, et al. Challenges with implementing the centers for disease control and prevention opioid guideline: a consensus panel report. Pain Med 2019;20:724–35.
3. Hooten WM. Chronic pain and mental health disorders: shared neural mechanisms, epidemiology, and treatment. Mayo Clin Proc 2016;91:955–70.
4. Garcia-Larrea L, Peyron R. Pain matrices and neuropathic pain matrices: a review. Pain 2013;154(Suppl 1):S29–43.
5. Pergolizzi JV Jr, LeQuang JA, Berger GK, et al. The basic pharmacology of opioids informs the opioid discourse about misuse and abuse: a review. Pain Ther 2017;6:1–16.
6. Stein C. Opioid receptors. Annu Rev Med 2016;67:433–51.
7. Ladapo JA, Larochelle MR, Chen A, et al. Physician prescribing of opioids to patients at increased risk of overdose from benzodiazepine use in the United States. JAMA Psychiatry 2018;75:623–30.
8. Jeffery MM, Hooten WM, Jena AB, et al. Rates of physician coprescribing of opioids and benzodiazepines after the release of the centers for disease control and prevention guidelines in 2016. JAMA Netw Open 2019;2:e198325.
9. Keller S, Bann CM, Dodd SL, et al. Validity of the brief pain inventory for use in documenting the outcomes of patients with noncancer pain. Clin J Pain 2004; 20:309–18.

10. Krebs EE, Lorenz KA, Bair MJ, et al. Development and initial validation of the PEG, a three-item scale assessing pain intensity and interference. J Gen Intern Med 2009;24:733–8.
11. Kroenke K, Spitzer RL, Williams JB. The patient health questionnaire-2: validity of a two-item depression screener. Med Care 2003;41:1284–92.
12. Kroenke K, Spitzer RL, Williams JB, et al. Anxiety disorders in primary care: prevalence, impairment, comorbidity, and detection. Ann Intern Med 2007;146: 317–25.
13. McNeely J, Wu LT, Subramaniam G, et al. Performance of the tobacco, alcohol, prescription medication, and other substance use (TAPS) tool for substance use screening in primary care patients. Ann Intern Med 2016;165:690–9.
14. National Institute on Drug Abuse. Tobacco, alcohol, prescription medication and other substance use tool. Availabl at: https://www.drugabuse.gov/taps/-/. Accessed January 20, 2020.
15. Jones T, Lookatch S, Moore T. Validation of a new risk assessment tool: the brief risk questionnaire. J Opioid Manag 2015;11:171–83.
16. Akbik H, Butler SF, Budman SH, et al. Validation and clinical application of the screener and opioid assessment for patients with pain (SOAPP). J Pain Symptom Manage 2006;32:287–93.
17. McAuliffe Staehler TM, Palombi LC. Beneficial opioid management strategies: a review of the evidence for the use of opioid treatment agreements. Subst Abus 2020;1–8 [Epub ahead of print].
18. Hooten WM. CAREFUL: a practical guide for improving the clinical surveillance of long-term opioid therapy. Mayo Clin Proc 2018;93:1149.
19. Brennan MJ. The effect of opioid therapy on endocrine function. Am J Med 2013; 126:S12–8.
20. Donegan D, Bancos I. Opioid-induced adrenal insufficiency. Mayo Clin Proc 2018;93:937–44.
21. Berna C, Kulich RJ, Rathmell JP. Tapering long-term opioid therapy in chronic noncancer pain: evidence and recommendations for everyday practice. Mayo Clin Proc 2015;90:828–42.
22. Centers for Disease Control and Prevention. Pocket guide: tapering opioids for chronic pain. Available at: https://www.cdc.gov/drugoverdose/prescribing/clinical-tools.html. Accessed January 20, 2020.
23. Demidenko MI, Dobscha SK, Morasco BJ, et al. Suicidal ideation and suicidal self-directed violence following clinician-initiated prescription opioid discontinuation among long-term opioid users. Gen Hosp Psychiatry 2017;47:29–35.
24. James JR, Scott JM, Klein JW, et al. Mortality after discontinuation of primary care-based chronic opioid therapy for pain: a retrospective cohort study. J Gen Intern Med 2019;34:2749–55.
25. Perez HR, Buonora M, Cunningham CO, et al. Opioid taper is associated with subsequent termination of care: a retrospective cohort study. J Gen Intern Med 2020;35:36–42.
26. Darnall BD, Ziadni MS, Stieg RL, et al. Patient-centered prescription opioid tapering in community outpatients with chronic pain. JAMA Intern Med 2018; 178:707–8.
27. Washington State Agency Medical Directors' Group. Interagency guideline on prescribing opioids for pain. 3rd edition 2015. Available at: http://www.agencymeddirectors.wa.gov/Files/2015AMDGOpioidGuideline.pdf. Accessed January 20, 2020.

28. Gowing L, Farrell M, Ali R, et al. Alpha(2)-adrenergic agonists for the management of opioid withdrawal. Cochrane Database Syst Rev 2016;(5):CD002024.
29. Fishman M, Tirado C, Alam D, et al. Safety and efficacy of lofexidine for medically managed opioid withdrawal: a randomized controlled clinical trial. J Addict Med 2019;13:169–76.
30. Salehi M, Kheirabadi GR, Maracy MR, et al. Importance of gabapentin dose in treatment of opioid withdrawal. J Clin Psychopharmacol 2011;31:593–6.
31. Pozzi G, Conte G, De Risio S. Combined use of trazodone-naltrexone versus clonidine-naltrexone in rapid withdrawal from methadone treatment. A comparative inpatient study. Drug Alcohol Depend 2000;59:287–94.
32. Mannelli P, Peindl K, Wu LT, et al. The combination very low-dose naltrexone-clonidine in the management of opioid withdrawal. Am J Drug Alcohol Abuse 2012;38:200–5.
33. White CM. Loperamide: a readily available but dangerous opioid substitute. J Clin Pharmacol 2019;59:1165–9.
34. Huffman KL, Rush TE, Fan Y, et al. Sustained improvements in pain, mood, function and opioid use post interdisciplinary pain rehabilitation in patients weaned from high and low dose chronic opioid therapy. Pain 2017;158:1380–94.
35. Frank JW, Lovejoy TI, Becker WC, et al. Patient outcomes in dose reduction or discontinuation of long-term opioid therapy: a systematic review. Ann Intern Med 2017;167:181–91.
36. Fishbain DA, Pulikal A. Does opioid tapering in chronic pain patients result in improved pain or same pain vs increased pain at taper completion? A structured evidence-based systematic review. Pain Med 2019;20:2179–97.

Ethics and Regulation of Opioid Prescriptions for Management of Pain
The Washington State Experience

James R. Babington, MD[a],*, Micah Matthews, MPA[b]

KEYWORDS

- Chronic pain • Opioid therapy • Ethics • Pain management • Health care regulation

KEY POINTS

- Discussion of the ethical decision making underpinning opioid therapy for non-malignant pain.
- Development of regulations regarding the provision of chronic opioid therapy for non-malignant pain.
- Importance of comprehensive interdisciplinary management to improve outcomes for patients suffering from non-malignant pain.

Pain is a ubiquitous human experience and essential to life itself. Its presence is one of the most common reasons to seek medical care.[1] The International Association for the Study of Pain (IASP) defines pain as "an unpleasant sensory and emotional experience associated with actual or potential tissue damage, or described in terms of such damage."[2] In 2016, the Centers for Disease Control and Prevention (CDC) analyzed the National Health Interview Survey data and estimated 20.4% (50.0 million) US adults had chronic pain and 8.0% (19.6 million) had high-impact chronic pain.[3] As such, medical providers are confronted daily with a symptom that results in significant morbidity and disability. The treatment of pain that arises from a clearly identifiable pathoanatomic lesion behaving in an expected manner is a satisfying demonstration of success in contemporary medical practice. However, the presence of pain that persists beyond the expected healing time or without a discreet pathoanatomic lesion continues to prove more problematic. Herein lies a more fundamental problem that has vexed physicians for millennia. Current biomedical assessment of pain relies on identifying an objective reason for pain, yet far too often we are bereft of a correctable

[a] Swedish Pain Services, Swedish Medical Center, 21616 76th Avenue West, Suite 212, Edmonds, WA 98026, USA; [b] Washington Medical Commission, 111 Israel Road Southeast, Tumwater, WA 98501, USA
* Corresponding author.
E-mail address: James.babington@swedish.org

Phys Med Rehabil Clin N Am 31 (2020) 279–287
https://doi.org/10.1016/j.pmr.2020.01.004
1047-9651/20/© 2020 Elsevier Inc. All rights reserved.

pathoanatomic diagnosis and rely on the "subjective" patient report. This evolving discourse leads to a fundamental undertreatment of pain and continues to be relevant to the discourse on pain today.[4]

Accepting that there is an evolving understanding of the human pain experience that does not appear to be coming to any clear conclusion at present, clinicians are rendering care to patients on a daily basis. The IASP has revised their classification of chronic pain to allow for further epidemiologic study and more discreet understanding of chronic pain.[5] The treatment of pain initially focuses on resolution of a pathoanatomic lesion. In the case that the painful condition cannot be remedied, care is focused on management of symptoms. The best evidence suggests that a multimodal, interdisciplinary approach to pain control may represent the most effective strategy to treating pain.[6] As a part of the multimodal approach, opioid therapy may play a role in symptom mitigation.

Derivatives of the opium poppy have been used since sometime around 3400 BCE and were referred to as *hul gil* by ancient Sumerians: the "joy plant." In the nineteenth century, German chemists developed morphine and diacetylmorphine (heroin) for therapeutic use.[7] Contemporary understanding of pain perception in mammals involves a ligand receptor model whereby endogenous and exogenous opioids act on μ-receptors, κ-receptors, and δ-receptors at spinal and supraspinal sites, which modulate signal transduction and intracellular processes.[8] Dopamine and opioid systems are postulated to contribute to both pain and pleasure.[9] This neurophysiologic behavior complicates the use of exogenous opioids for therapeutic purposes. Although this relationship allows opioids to relieve pain, it carries the risk of substance misuse and dependence. Moreover, opioids interact in other deleterious ways that can involve increased fracture risk, mental health concerns, respiratory arrest, and death.[10,11]

There is a conflicting understanding about the utility of chronic exposure to opioids. Not all humans exposed to opioids will escalate or misuse the substance, nor will they suffer the very severe consequences of fatal overdose. Clinicians routinely observe that some patients respond favorably to opioids, although long-term evidence of benefit is still being elucidated.[12,13] Some argue that low-dose, structured, and highly monitored opioid therapy may be beneficial.[14] Recently published data suggest that long-term opioid therapy can be considered in well-selected and monitored patients suffering from osteoarthritis, diabetic peripheral neuropathy, and chronic low-back pain.[15] The therapeutic utility of opioids is an area of intense debate in the literature without a clear clinical consensus.

It is within this context that providers are faced with the ethical dilemma of using a substance with significant known risks and therapeutic benefit in treating noncancer chronic pain with opioid therapy. As the "opioid crisis" evolves in the United States, physicians need to determine when and if opioids can be used safely in an individual patient with conflicting data on efficacy while navigating the backdrop of a public health crisis with limited alternatives that are routinely funded by insurers. The public health concern commonly described as the "opioid crisis" often conflates the legitimate use of prescription opioids with the misuse of the same substances and the illicit drug trade. The data regarding prescriptions of opioids after implementation of prescription monitoring programs demonstrate a curtailment by 30% of schedule II opioids and presumed more appropriate use of opioid therapy.[16] Often when data are presented to shape physician and policy-making behavior, little is done that clearly helps distinguish between opioids coming from prescription use for legitimate pain concerns versus nonprescribed use of prescription versus illicit heroin- or fentanyl-containing substances.

The Hippocratic tradition and its principle-based subsequent formulations create an ethical duty on the part of the physician to relieve suffering to the individual patient's benefit.[17] This deontological approach applies an overarching principle-based deductive reasoning to a clinical situation. Although this line of thought supports more global ideas, such as "if a patient seeks out a physician's care, then the physician is obliged to provide treatment in the patient's best interest," it becomes more challenging to use such a principle-based approach when dealing with opioid therapy because so little is known about both the disease and its treatment.

Inductive reasoning, which creates a valid argument based on strength of the premises, seems more applicable in the clinical situation whereby there are few known absolute truths. Rather, there is a multitude of clinical situations with variable degrees of strength. Using the framework of Beauchamp and Childress[18] for ethical decision making can prove helpful in determining when and how physicians should evaluate treatment options. That framework focuses on providing care that respects patient autonomy, minimizes harm (nonmaleficence), maximizes benefit (beneficence), and ensures justice. Cohen and Jangro[19] argue that such a case-based approach is necessary in providing an ethical framework for the application of opioid therapy.

The paternalistic, traditional model of the doctor-patient relationship has been supplanted predominantly by a guidance-cooperation model.[20] This model empowers patients in decision making while creating a dilemma for the provider with prescriptive authority for a controlled substance. Using classical deontological approaches, one might feel compelled to provide the opioid upon the patient's request. Ballantyne and Fleischer[21] present conditions, particularly when a clinician judges a treatment will do more harm than good, when there is no obligation to provide treatment and the patient has no right to demand it; thus, the physician is ethically justified to refuse opioid therapy.

The physician's primary duty is to the individual patient. However, the use of opioids for therapeutic purposes has created a conflict in the midst of a public health crisis involving opioid misuse. It was in this setting that legislators in Washington State called for rule making regarding the therapeutic use of opioids. The collaboration between the legislators, regulators, and prescribers created a set of prescribing rules that created a framework to help guide prescriber behavior. This kind of collaboration is essential to ensure the interests of the community while preserving the patient-physician relationship and physician ethical duties, and creating an environment that allows physicians and patients to safely decide when and if opioids can be therapeutically used based on the science available.

Perhaps some of the most unnecessarily feared words in the English lexicon are "I am from the government and I am here to help." A more prudent concern may be the law or directive behind the presence of the regulator. In the case of the opioid-prescribing rules adopted by the Washington Medical Commission (WMC), which governs the practice of medicine of allopathic physicians and physician assistants, and the 4 other prescribing regulatory boards (Board of Osteopathic Medicine and Surgery, Board of Podiatric Medicine, Nursing Care Quality Assurance Commission, and Board of Pharmacy) in 2018/2019, the intent and directive did not actually come from the regulator but instead from the Legislature with affirmation by the Governor. With such a divided origin, it is difficult to concisely state the intent of the rules. One can surmise that the elected officials desired to be on the record-taking decisive action in light of growing use and misuse of opioids and the sometimes fatal sequelae. Political commitment to the issue is appreciated by those regulators that must carry out directives, but a known danger arises when those unfamiliar with the intricacies of an issue, such as elected officials, attempt to be proscriptive in their fix.

It was at this point that the professional associations and the regulatory bodies intervened in the 2017 legislative process to advocate for general rule-making authority to address the newly declared crisis. The request for rule-making authority was in response to the numerous and restrictive bills being considered that would give practitioners few options and little to no room for discretion. Put another way, the regulators and associations told the elected officials that they recognized and understood the problem, but for the good of patients and prescribers, please leave the details to those who actually practice and regulate medicine. From this arose collaboration between professional associations and state regulators to devise clinically appropriate rules regarding the prescription of opioids for therapeutic purposes. The WMC is made up of 21 Governor Appointees: 6 public members, 2 physician assistants, and 13 physicians of various specialties. These commissioners make the legally mandated decisions on licensing, discipline, and creating rules.

From the regulatory perspective, the strategy behind the work at WMC is risk based or through the nudge approach. Essentially, the approach is to take the minimum action necessary to encourage positive behavior change. For example, a patient with an acute injury receiving an opioid prescription might not be concerning, but if that patient comes back for another 7-day prescription refill, there should be concern that healing is not progressing as expected or there may be other concerns. Therefore, a mandated check of the Prescription Monitoring Program (PMP) was included as part of the regulation. The PMP in Washington State is a statewide data repository of Drug Enforcement Administration scheduled therapeutic agents that can be accessed by all licensed prescribers and records opioids prescribed and dispensed to a particular patient. Those kinds of behavioral reminders or nudges are placed strategically throughout the rules. Finally, it had to be clear that an administrative rule adopted by the WMC needs to represent the floor of acceptable medical practice and not the ceiling. That final point was exceptionally difficult for some stakeholders to accept.

The WMC defined the scope as relating to the 4 pain phases (acute operative and nonoperative, subacute, and chronic), coprescribing of benzodiazepines, and prescription monitoring requirements for practitioners. These areas of focus were largely determined based on current evidence, trends in case law, and interest by the public, practitioners, and elected officials.

The patients with acute operative and nonoperative pain have had an injury or surgery that recently occurred. The rules do not mandate but recommend no more than a 3-day prescription of opioid therapy and not prescribe beyond a 7-day supply (acute nonoperative) or 14-day supply for acute perioperative pain without clinical documentation to justify the needs for such a quantity. Upon reevaluation, the prescriber can extend the duration of an opioid prescription to provide the patient with the care they need based on documented rational medical decision making.

If a patient has received opioids for more than 6 weeks, they enter the subacute category. The patient receiving opioids for more than 31 days and 700 morphine equivalent dose cumulative dose are at higher risk for needing long-term opioid therapy.[22] The WMC made the decision to leave the chronic pain prescribing rules largely unchanged from the 2011 format. The maintenance of the chronic pain rules was in response to members of the chronic pain community providing their feedback throughout the process, which was greatly appreciated. The initial set of rulemaking by the WMC in 2012 had robust risk assessment and monitoring for this group of patients.

Two significant additional nudges were added in the section regulating prescribing opioid therapy for more than 12 weeks and in the chronic category. The first directs the practitioner to completely reevaluate the patient as if presenting with a new disease if they progress from the subacute to chronic phase, that is, remain on opioids for more than 12 weeks. The second is the addition of the grace period or safe harbor for taking on new chronic pain patients and evaluating their current treatment regimen against function and quality of life. The intent of these rules is to encourage more consideration on the part of practitioners to thoroughly evaluate the patient suffering from chronic pain and develop a comprehensive risk-based approach to development of their treatment plan.

An unintended consequence of these rules has been a reluctance of providers to continue to manage long-term opioid therapy because of fear of regulatory repercussions. Clinically, there has been a growing number of providers who "don't do pain" and who refuse to prescribe opioids in any form, and who are expeditiously tapering patients managed on long-term opioid therapy to arbitrary morphine equivalent goals based on misinterpretation of guidelines put forth by the CDC and Food and Drug Administration (FDA). Rapid taper or non-provision of opioid therapy has been compounded by large Washington State health systems unilaterally declaring all of their covered patients will be tapered below a morphine milligram equivalent (MME) without consideration of function, quality of life, or provision of supported tapers, which have shown benefit in successfully tapering patients receiving chronic opioid therapy.[23] The MME chosen can range from 90 MME or as low as 50 MME. These MME levels, well below the consultation threshold in place since 2012, and the refusal to coprescribe certain medications with opioid therapy represent a questionable risk profile on the part of the health system that seems to embrace removing practitioner discretion and will leave legitimate pain patients in significantly disrupted lifestyles without any support or treatment directed toward managing chronic pain. There is evidence that abrupt and unsupported opioid cessation can result in adverse health outcomes.[24] It is also entirely possible these seemingly extreme postures by health systems may lead to increased suicidal behavior in these already compromised patient populations.[25] In response, the Washington State Department of Health, the WMC, CDC, Health and Human Services, and FDA have all issued clarifying statements suggesting that a thorough evaluation of the patient and the appropriateness of therapy are essential rather than a fear-based response to possible regulatory oversight.[26,27] This thoughtful approach to care is the intent of the regulators in Washington State and of significant importance as a rising tide of patient harm emerges in the data regarding rapid deescalation of opioids in patients on long-term opioid therapy.[28]

In making the rules, the primary goal of the WMC is transparency. To that end, 7 meetings were held around the state to gather input from the public, practitioners, state experts, and anyone else who chose to participate. Hundreds of written comments were received, each of which received a response in an open public meeting. Many comments were acted on and resulted in alteration of the rules.

The second goal gets to the heart of this article, balance: how does one approach a regulatory assignment that is so broad and impactful while still meeting the needs of all of the stakeholders? To answer briefly, with confidence and extreme care. There is a certain level of outward confidence required to practice the art of medicine. Regulators must possess a similar level of confidence. One must have respect for the effort it takes to enter the profession and the diligence required to maintain the practice. One must assume a positive intent on the part of practitioners and that they simply want to practice good medicine. The positive intention on the part of the practioner is what should dictate how one crafts rules and policies: enable practitioners to practice their art, correct when the needs arise, and hold accountable when required. Perhaps most of all, one must have the confidence to know that one is capable of doing the right thing.

In formulating the rules, the WMC was mandated to consider guidelines from the CDC and the Agency Medical Directors Group (AMDG) to frame the debate within a short timeline. The CDC and AMDG guidelines were not considered documents that established a floor of acceptable treatment. The years 2017 to 2019 also represented the time period in which many people were either questioning or misapplying the CDC guidelines to the detriment of patients, specifically with regard to tapering. In order to accommodate the floor-to-ceiling debate, the WMC attempted to preserve practitioner discretion in the rules and did not establish hard pill limits for any pain phase, only recommendations.

This decision to not place specific pill limits was vocally protested by the offices of several statewide elected officials as well as 1 member of the Opioid Joint Task Force. The Task Force took this position despite political pressure because it created a regulatory environment that allowed for appropriate use of opioids to treat patients suffering from chronic pain and preserved the ability of prescribers to practice medicine within the current state of knowledge. On 3 separate occasions, this group of political appointees took a principled stand against powerful influences to protect the ability to provide appropriate care to patients.

In the end, the rules were adopted on time, and the WMC chose to not make them effective for the maximum allowable time so education efforts in concert with the medical association could be undertaken. However, such a forced rush did provide learning opportunities, the first of which was an oversight relating to the definition of a hospital, and whether long-term acute care centers or skilled nursing facilities would be excluded from parts of the rule. The WMC's intent was that long-term acute care centers and skilled nursing facilities would be treated the same as in-patient hospital settings and excluded, but the rule was not explicitly clear. The confusion regarding the definition of a hospital resulted in a hasty interpretive statement being adopted to clarify the issue. There are several other clean-up items needed that have resulted in the reopening of the rules in order to address the new legislative requirements from 2019. Perhaps the most complex item that may not be possible for the WMC to address in its rules because of scope and jurisdiction issues is the influence of multiple third parties in the patient-practitioner relationship. From chain pharmacy partial fill policies to benefit managers and prior authorization to state Medicaid payment policies, these influences are more often attempts to supplant the will of the practitioner and the choice of the patient, often with little legal basis or consensus. Although the WMC may not be able to address these issues through the Medical Practice Act, the organization is certainly interested in collaboration to solve these barriers to patient care and practitioner discretion.

The second lesson was not successfully advocating for a longer timeline for education regarding implementations. There are major medical groups, that, even a year after the implementation date of the prescribing rules, are still not entirely compliant. The failure to fully comply with the rule lies in a complex medical system in an age of consolidation and electronic medical records, which requires time-intensive changes to workflows in order to adapt to these new requirements. Although the WMC did not have as much time for education as hoped, the WMC did stretch the legal mandate to the breaking point, provided comprehensive continuing medical education, and engaged physician partners throughout the state to emphasize educational efforts to assist providers in reaching the standards set forth in the rules.

The third and perhaps most significant learning was adopting too collaborative a tone and posture during the initial rule-making phases. Washington State had 5 regulatory boards and commissions required to make rules. At 34,000, the WMC regulates the most prescribers in Washington State with an easy second going to the Nursing Commission. In an effort to lead to a more unified rule-making process, the WMC took a position of collaboration: allowing the Department of Health to take the lead on the initial effort of writing prescribing rules. The lesson for others looking to tackle this endeavor is to come to the most consistent rules by allowing the stakeholders and regulators who have the most direct authority to lead the rule-making process.

The decision to have the Department of Health draft the initial template rules resulted in unnecessary inclusions. It also resulted in a less than productive feedback model and stunted progress during the open meeting portion of the project. Finally, because of this rule-making structure, the individual regulatory bodies adopted differing standards or requirements in the final rules, which is precisely what everyone wanted to avoid by being collaborative in the process. It should be noted that the WMC acted on the error early and began meeting separately to develop its own rules draft, which were brought to the full Opioid Joint Task Force and largely adopted. The rule making was done in collaboration with the state medical association and patient advocacy groups. Although resulting in a better outcome, it is likely poor consolation for those that are negatively impacted on a system level.

Although the individual regulators adopted what they thought were profession-specific and possibly minor changes, the end result is the same: inconsistency introduced in the final hour in key areas of the rules that must be reckoned with at the practice level. The adoption of disparate rules by each of the boards and commissions has resulted in confusion and frustration for clinicians, most notably in those working in larger health systems, where the more restrictive rule standards have been applied to all prescribers to ease compliance concerns. It is doubly frustrating for WMC members and staff whose intent was to create rules containing practitioner discretion, only to have that discretion removed by application of more restrictive standards by systems.

Every action of significance taken by a regulatory body, no matter how studied, results in an unintended consequence. Were these rules ideal? Definitely not. However, one must remember that these were the years that state attorneys general were charging prescribers as criminals for what used to be medical practice. The US Department of Justice was becoming more interested in state regulatory enforcement actions as a basis for their cases, and politicians decried the unacceptable level of overdose deaths "in our neighborhoods" despite the fact that death and addiction were far from a new concept in communities of color. As stated at a national tri-regulator symposium in 2015, "This is not a new problem, it is just new that the victims are white and middle class."

In viewing the rules through that lens, were they ideal? Rules never are. Are they the right tool to establish a floor for acceptable practice to protect patients? Absolutely. Were they necessary to avoid a greater harm imposed on practitioners? Clearly. Would the WMC advocate for the rules as a solution again? Without hesitation; if for no better reason than experience says not to trust anyone other than practitioners to arrive at the most correct solution for clinical practice and patient safety. "Act only according to that maxim whereby you can at the same time will that it should become a universal law" (Immanuel Kant, Categorial Imperative).

Although no deontologic ethic underlies the use of opioids, a deductively valid deontology supports the physician treatment of patient's pain. The Kantian categorical imperative supports the fact that all patients should be treated with dignity and respect. By recognizing that pain, particularly long-term pain, defies many of the precepts of a model focused on cure of a pathoanatomic lesion, a case-based ethic will be necessary to determine treatment plans. The decision to use or not to use opioids should remain firmly within the purview of the physician-patient dyad with a focus on safety and appropriate use. Regulation developed collaboratively between physicians and regulators can help to protect the public good and allow physicians to focus their attention on the appropriate application of opioids in individual cases.

Ultimately, persistent pain will continue to defy many of the medical models. To effectively provide care for patients, access will need to include interdisciplinary strategies for the treatment of long-term pain. Years of simplistic treatment of pain with opioid therapy have created a cohort of patients for whom opioid therapy has been a mainstay of treatment. Forced and expeditious tapering of these individuals without any support raises serious ethical and medical concerns. Regulatory oversight can help create a framework for providing appropriate care of patients with opioid therapy. Evolving models of care for patients suffering from persistent pain must include more comprehensive methods, including interdisciplinary care and addressing the deleterious effects of chronic exposure to high-potency opioids. From a policy perspective, this will ultimately require rethinking how pain is conceptualized and transcend the current fee-for-service models. Going forward, collaboration between all the stakeholders: physicians, patients, regulators, pharmaceutical manufacturers, health systems, insurers, and politicians, is essential to ensure that the highest-quality appropriate care is funded.

DISCLOSURE

Neither author has any commercial or financial conflicts of interest or any external funding sources.

REFERENCES

1. Schappert SM, Burt CW. Ambulatory care visits to physician offices, hospital outpatient departments, and emergency departments: United States, 2001-02. Vital Health Stat 13 2006;(159):1–66.
2. Merskey H, Lindblom U, Mumford JM, et al. Classification of chronic pain. In: Merskey H, Bogduk N, editors. IASP task force on taxonomy. 2nd edition. Seattle (WA): IASP Press; 1994. p. 209–14.
3. Dahlhamer J, Lucas J, Zelaya C, et al. Prevalence of chronic pain and high-impact chronic pain among adults–United States, 2016. MMWR Morb Mortal Wkly Rep 2018;67(36):1001–6.
4. Goldberg DS. The bioethics of pain management beyond opioids. New York: Routledge. Taylor and Francis; 2014.
5. Treede RD, Rief W, Barke A, et al. Chronic pain as a symptom or a disease: the IASP classification of chronic pain for the International Classification of Diseases (ICD-11). Pain 2019;160:19–27.
6. Flor H, Fydrich T, Turk DC. Efficacy of multidisciplinary pain treatment centers: a meta-analytic review. Pain 1992;49(2):221–30.
7. Bandyopadhyay S. An 8,000-year history of use and abuse of opium and opioids: how that matters for a successful control of the epidemic? Neurology 2019;92(15 supplement):4–9, 055.
8. Kanjhan R. Opioids and pain. Clin Exp Pharmacol Physiol 1995;22(6–7):397–403.
9. Leknes S, Tracey I. A common neurobiology for pain and pleasure. Nat Rev Neurosci 2008;9:314–20.
10. Ray W, Chung CP, Murray KT, et al. Prescription of long-acting opioids and mortality in patients with noncancer pain. JAMA 2016;315(22):2415–23.
11. Chou R, Turner JA, Devine EB, et al. The effectiveness and risks of long-term opioid therapy for chronic pain: a systematic review for a National Institutes of Health Pathways to Prevention Workshop. Ann Intern Med 2015;1624:276–86.

12. Portenoy RK. Opioid therapy for chronic nonmalignant pain: clinicians' perspective. J Law Med Ethics 1996;24(4):296–309.

13. Cowan DT, Wilson-Barnett J, Griffiths P, et al. A randomized, double-blind, placebo-controlled, crossover pilot study to assess the effects of long-term opioid drug consumption and subsequent abstinence in chronic non-cancer pain patients receiving controlled-release morphine. Pain Med 2005;6:113–4.

14. Ballantyne JC. Opioids for chronic nonterminal pain. South Med J 2006;99(11): 1245–55.

15. Bialas P, Maier C, Klose P, et al. Efficacy and harms of long-term opioid therapy in chronic non-cancer pain: systematic review and meta-analysis of open-label extension trials with a study duration > 26 weeks. Eur J Pain 2020;24(2):265–78.

16. Bao Y, Pan Y, Taylor A, et al. Prescription drug monitoring programs are associated with sustained reductions in opioid prescribing by physicians. Health Aff 2016;35(6):1045–51.

17. Antoniou SA, Antoniou GA, Granderath FA, et al. Reflections of the Hippocratic Oath in modern medicine. World J Surg 2010;34(12):3075–9.

18. Beauchamp T, Childress J. Principles of biomedical ethics. 7th edition. New York: Oxford University Press; 2012.

19. Cohen MJ, Jangro WC. A clinical ethics approach to opioid treatment of chronic non cancer pain. AMA J Ethics 2015;17(6):521–9.

20. Szaz T, Hollender J. The basic model of the doctor-patients relationship. Arch Intern Med 1956;97:85–90.

21. Ballantyne JC, Fleischer LA. Ethical issues in opioid prescribing for chronic pain. Pain 2010;148(3):365–7.

22. Shah A, Hayes CJ, Martin BC. Characteristics of initial prescription episodes and likelihood of long-term opioid use–United States, 2006-2015. MMWR Morb Mortal Wkly Rep 2017;66(10):265–9.

23. Sullivan MD, Turner JA, DiLodovico C, et al. Prescription opioid taper support for outpatients with chronic pain: a randomized controlled trial. J Pain 2017;18(3): 308–18.

24. Mark TL, Parish W. Opioid medication discontinuation and risk of adverse opioid-related health care events. J Subst Abuse Treat 2019;103:58–63.

25. Cheatle MD. Depression, chronic pain, and suicide by overdose: on the edge. Pain Med 2011;12(suppl 2):S43–8.

26. Lofy K, Roberts AW, Rude TD, et al. Clarification of opioid prescribing rules. Olympia: Department of Health State of Washington; 2019. Available at: https://wmc.wa. gov/sites/default/files/public/documents/Clarification-opioid-rules_9-20-2019.pdf.

27. HHS Guide for clinicians on the appropriate dosage reduction or discontinuation of long-term opioid analgesics. Available at: https://www.hhs.gov/opioids/sites/ default/files/2019-10/Dosage_Reduction_Discontinuation.pdf.

28. Mackey K, Anderson J, Bourne D, et al. Evidence brief: benefits and harms of long-term opioid dose reduction or discontinuation in patients with chronic pain. Washington, DC: Evidence Synthesis Program, Health Services Research and Development Service, Office of Research and Development, Department of Veterans Affairs; 2019. VA ESP Project #09-199; Available at: https://www. hsrd.research.va.gov/publications/esp/reports.cfm.

Opioids
Pharmacology, Physiology, and Clinical Implications in Pain Medicine

Andrew Friedman, MD[a,b,*], Lorifel Nabong, PharmD, BCACP[c]

KEYWORDS

- Opioids • Pharmacology • Physiology • Pain management

KEY POINTS

- Opioids regulate human responses to pain and stress as well as reward in humans through interrelated mechanisms.
- Recent research has clarified the specific risks and benefits of opioids in chronic pain management.
- Key aspects of pharmacology related to the medical use of opioids are reviewed.

INTRODUCTION

Opioid receptors and opioid agonists are widespread throughout nature. Endogenous opioids mediate complex functions in animals and in humans. The opioid system in humans plays a central role in pain control and is a key mediator of hedonic homeostasis, mood, and well-being. This system also regulates responses to stress and several peripheral physiologic functions, including respiratory, gastrointestinal, endocrine, and immune systems. The use of opioid medicine in the management of chronic pain has become increasingly controversial. This article provides an overview of the basic physiology of opioids, reviews opioid pharmacology, and attempts to address several issues of current importance in the management of patients with established long-term opioid therapy.

HISTORY

Opium contains a mix of opioid alkaloids, including morphine and codeine, and has been used since prehistory. Its use developed in the Middle East, and evidence of

[a] Physical Medicine and Rehabilitation, Virginia Mason Medical Center, 1100 9th Avenue, Seattle, WA 98111, USA; [b] University of WA, Seattle, WA, USA; [c] Virginia Mason Medical Center, 1100 9th Avenue, Seattle, WA 98111, USA
* Corresponding author. Physical Medicine and Rehabiliation, Virginia Mason Medical Center, 1100 9th Avenue, Seattle, WA 98111.
E-mail address: Andrew.friedman@virginiamason.org

Phys Med Rehabil Clin N Am 31 (2020) 289–303
https://doi.org/10.1016/j.pmr.2020.01.007
1047-9651/20/© 2020 Elsevier Inc. All rights reserved.

pmr.theclinics.com

cultivation of opium poppies has been found in tombs in Egypt and Mesopotamia. Greek physicians were aware of its medicinal properties as early as 1500 BCE. It is thought that Arab traders brought opium to China and India around 800 CE, and it subsequently found its way to all parts of Europe by around 1300.[1] In countries where opium is indigenously consumed, doses of between 75 and 3000 morphine equivalents (MED) daily appear to be common when the drug is smoked.[2]

Morphine was first synthesized in Germany in 1804. Codeine was isolated a few years later, followed by hydrocodone and hydromorphone. Diacetyl morphine, or heroin, was introduced in 1898.[3] Methadone was synthesized in 1939 and oxycodone in 1916. Buprenorphine was developed in the 1970s. Controlled release oxycodone was approved by the Food and Drug Administration in 1995 and entered the US market in 1996.[4]

PHYSIOLOGY

Opioid receptors are a type of G protein–coupled receptor distributed widely in the central and peripheral nervous system of vertebrates, including humans. Three types of opioid receptors, mu, delta, and kappa, were discovered in the 1970s. They share a highly conserved transmembrane structure but differ significantly in both extracellular and intracellular structure and are thought to have significantly different but closely interrelated functions.[5]

The mu opioid receptor was named after it was found to be the primary binding site for morphine. Mu opioid receptors mediate the antinociceptive properties of opioids as well as the rewarding aspects of nonopioid drugs of abuse, including cannabinoids, alcohol, and nicotine, as well as the reward of such activities as social interaction. These receptors are found in high density in supraspinal locations, primarily at presynaptic sites, and generally inactivate ascending pathways and activate descending pathways. They are found in high concentration in the limbic system and in areas of the brain associated with neurohormonal secretion, such as in the hypothalamus. In addition to the functions mentioned above, mu receptors have important functions in the modulation of responses to pain and stress.[5] The mu receptor is the primary target for most current opioid agonists used to treat pain.

The primary endogenous opioid acting at the mu receptor is beta endorphin. Beta endorphin is a peptide produced from the precursor peptide proopioomelanocortin (POMC). POMC is produced in the hypothalamus, an area rich in systems mediating not only reward, satiation, and pain but also hormonal systems regulating the pituitary and adrenal axis. POMC is cleaved to produce not only beta endorphin but also adrenocorticotrophic hormone, a primary stress hormone. Responses to stress and pain are closely interrelated.

Human endogenous opioid systems are highly homeostatic. For example, in the production of POMC, its products beta endorphin and corticotropin are reduced in the setting of chronic opioid exposure and chronic stress hormone exposure. It is also understood that states of chronic stress may induce tolerance to endogenous opioids and subsequently poorer internal pain regulation via changes in the mu receptor system.

Kappa opioid receptors are thought to mediate distinct physiologic processes when compared with the mu receptor. They are found in higher density in the spinal cord and thought to have a significant role in the production of hyperalgesia. Kappa receptors have been thought to be important in the modulation of visceral pain. However, kappa agonists trialed to date have been found to be strongly dysphoric, a feature that has limited drug development to date.[6]

The third type of opioid receptor is the delta receptor. Compared with mu receptors, delta opioid receptors are found in relatively low concentrations in the midbrain but at high density in the dorsal root ganglia of peripheral nerves. They have a relatively low impact on acute pain perception but may have a more substantial role modulating chronic pain and nociception in the periphery and are a target for current pharmacologic research.[7] The primary endogenous agonist for delta receptors are the enkephalins, which are produced in the gut, sympathetic nervous system, and adrenal glands.

PHARMACOLOGY

The primary pharmacologic considerations of interest are absorption, distribution, metabolism, and excretion. All of these are of potential importance in the clinical use of opioids.

Absorption

Although there are a plethora of administration routes for opioid medications, oral and transdermal are the most commonly used,[8] followed by intravenous, intramuscular, and subcutaneous depending on practice setting (inpatient vs outpatient). Oral doses of opioids undergo hepatic first-pass metabolism, which can lead to individual variability of dose, therapeutic effect, and adverse effects. Of the oral medications, oxycodone and codeine have a reduced first-pass metabolism, thus allowing for more bioavailability as compared with other oral opioids. Morphine, on the other hand, is highly extracted by the liver; thus, oral bioavailability is approximately 33%. To minimize variability from first-pass metabolism, other routes, such as nasal, intravenous, sublingual/buccal, transdermal, and rectal, can be used. In general, the most common clinical indication for routes other than oral are intolerance of oral intake or alterations in gastrointestinal anatomy or function. For example, patients receiving chemotherapy and experiencing nausea and vomiting may consider alternative route of administration for opioid, such as intravenous, rectal, or buccal, which may also reduce potential for first-pass metabolism.[9] Caution is advised in contemplating equianalgesic doses in situations such as the one described because these equianalgesic doses may vary between individuals and incomplete cross-tolerance to different opioids is thought to exist.

Distribution

The analgesic effect of opioids results from interaction with mu, kappa, and delta opioid receptors found on neuronal membranes. However, in order for opioid medications to reach these neuronal membranes, tissue distribution is an important consideration (**Table 1**). All opioids bind to plasma protein, although with varying affinity. Once they are unbound, they leave the blood and localize in highly perfused tissues, such as brain, lung, kidney, and spleen. Distribution to various tissues is affected by physiologic and chemical factors. Lipophilicity is an important consideration. Morphine may have difficulty crossing the blood-brain barrier (BBB) because it is poorly lipophilic, whereas fentanyl, which is highly lipophilic, can cross easily. Pharmacodynamic effects influence more than tissue concentrations. For example, although morphine and fentanyl have similar half-lives, the physiologic effects of morphine in the central nervous system (CNS) are prolonged because it takes longer to cross over the BBB and also to exit the CNS through the BBB. Thus, morphine's nervous system effects last longer than those of fentanyl, which can quickly cross into and exit out of the CNS[9–11] (**Table 2**).

Table 1
Opioid receptor effects

Generic Name	Receptor Effects[a] μ	δ	κ	Approximately Equivalent Dose (mg)	Oral:Parenteral Potency Ratio	Duration of Analgesia (h)	Maximum Efficacy
Morphine[b]	+++	+		10	Low	4–5	High
Hydromorphone	+++			1.5	Low	4–5	High
Oxymorphone	+++			1.5	Low	3–4	High
Methadone	+++			10[c]	High	4–6	High
Meperidine	+++			60–100	Medium	2–4	High
Fentanyl	+++			0.1	Low	1–1.5	High
Sufentanil	+++	+	+	0.02	Parenteral only	1–1.5	High
Alfentanil	+++			Titrated	Parenteral only	0.25–0.75	High
Remifentanil	+++			Titrated[d]	Parenteral only	0.05[e]	High
Levorphanol	+++			2–3	High	4–5	High
Codeine	±			30–60	High	3–4	Low
Hydrocodone[f]	±			5–10	Medium	4–6	Moderate
Oxycodone[b,g]	++			4.5	Medium	3–4	Mod High
Pentazocine	±		+	30–50	Medium	3–4	Moderate
Nalbuphine	–		++	10	Parenteral only	3–6	High
Buprenorphine	±	–	–	0.3	Low	4–8	High
Butorphanol	±		+++	2	Parenteral only	3–4	High

[a] +++, ++, +, strong agonist; ±, partial or weak agonist; –, antagonist.
[b] Available in sustained-release forms, morphine (MS Contin); oxycodone (OxyCONTIN).
[c] No consensus, may have higher potency.
[d] Administered as an infusion at 0.025 to 0.2 μg/kg/min.
[e] Duration is dependent on a context-sensitive half-time of 3 to 4 min.
[f] Available in tablets containing acetaminophen (Norco, Vicodin, Lortab, others).
[g] Available in tablets containing acetaminophen (Percocet); aspirin (Percodan).
From Schumacher M, Basbaum A, Naidu R: Opioid analgesics and antagonists. In: Katzung BG, Trevor AJ eds. Basic and Clinical Pharmacology. 11th ed. New York, NY: McGraw-Hill, 2009:531-552; with permission.

Metabolism

Universally, the goal of drug metabolism is to covert a drug into a hydrophilic state to allow its excretion in the urine. Most of the metabolization of opioid takes place in the liver.

Phase I involves CYP450 enzymes (via oxidation or hydrolysis) and phase 2 involves metabolism by conjugation (ie, conjugate glucuronic acid, glycine, sulfate). In phase I, primary CYP enzymes include CYP3A4 and CYP2D6. Other important enzymes involved with opioid metabolism include CYP2C19, CYP2C9, CYP2C8, and CYP2B6, which are all required for methadone metabolism. Phase I metabolism is vital to bring on activation of analgesic effects of prodrugs, such as hydrocodone, tramadol, and codeine.[12]

Drug-drug interactions are primarily modulated by influences another drug may have on CYP3A4 and CYP2D6 enzymes. If the medication involved is a substrate, inhibitor, or inducer, it may influence clinical effects of the second drug. **Tables 2** elaborate the potential effects of CYP3A4/2D6 modulation on opioid pharmacokinetics and the effects on specific opioids.[9] A medication that is considered an

Table 2
Metabolic pathway/enzyme involvement

Opioid	Phase 1 Metabolism	Phase 2 Metabolism	Comment
Morphine[11]	None	Glucuronidation via UGT2B7	
Codeine[12]	CYP2D6	None	
Hydrocodone[13]	CYP2D6	None	One of the metabolites of hydrocodone is hydromorphone, which undergoes phase 2 glucuronidation
Oxycodone[10]	CYP3A4 CYP2D6	None	Oxycodone produces a small amount of oxymorphone, which must undergo subsequent metabolism via glucuronidation
Methadone[14]	CYP3A4 CYP2B6 CYP2C8 CYP2C19 CYP2D6 CYP2C9	None	CYP3A4 and CYP2B6 are the primary enzymes involved in methadone metabolism; other enzymes play a relatively minor role
Tramadol[15]	CYP3A4 CYP2D6	None	
Fentanyl[9]	CYP3A4	None	
Hydromorphone[16]	None	Glucuronidation via UGT2B7	
Oxymorphone[17]	None	Glucuronidation via UGT2B7	

From Smith HS. Opioid metabolism. Mayo Clin Proc. 2009;84(7):613-624; with permission.

inhibitor, is a drug that decreases activity of enzyme in CYP450 family, thus reducing metabolism of affected substrates. An inducer is a medication that increases activity of particular CYP enzyme and thus increases metabolism of substrate affected by the enzyme.[11]

As for phase II, glucuronidation is one of the most important phase II reactions. Glucuronidation is catalyzed by the enzyme uridine diphosphate glucuronosyltransferase (UGT) to develop highly polarized/hydrophilic drugs. The primary enzymes involved with glucuronidation of opioid medications are primarily UGT2B7 and UGT1A3 (hydrocodone and hydromorphone).[11,13]

Medications that only undergo phase II metabolism (morphine, hydromorphone, oxymorphone) have minimal drug-drug interactions as compared with counterparts that undergo phase I metabolism as well. These medications may be best considered in patients with significant polypharmacy, to reduce potential for drug-drug interactions[11-13] (**Table 3**).

Excretion

Excretion of polar opioid metabolites as well as small amounts of the parent drug is primarily in the urine. Caution must be taken for patients with poor renal function, especially for drugs with metabolites that are active after processing in the liver. In patients with renal dysfunction, medications, such as meperidine

Table 3 Major opioid metabolites			
Opioid	Inactive Metabolites	Active Metabolites Identical to Pharmaceutical Opioids	Active Metabolites that Are Not Pharmaceutical Opioids
Morphine[27]	Normorphine	Hydromorphone[a]	Morphone-3-G glucuronide Morphone-6-G glucuronide
Hydromorphone[16]	Minor metabolites	None	Hydromorphone-3-glucuronide
Hydrocodone	Norhydrocodone	Hydromorphone	None
Codeine	Norcodeine	Hydrocodone[a] Morphine	None
Oxycodone[10]	None	Oxymorphone	Noroxycodone
Oxymorphone[17]	Oxymorphone-3-glucuronide	None	6-Hydroxy-oxymorphone
Fentanyl[9]	Norfentanyl	None	None
Tramadol[15]	Nortramadol	None	O-desmethyltramadol
Methadone	2-Ethylidene-1,5-dimethyl-3,3-diphenylpyrrolidine 2-Ethyl-5-methyl-3,3-diphenylpyrroline	None	None
Heroin	Normorphine	Morphine	6-Monoacetylmorphine

[a] Only very low levels are seen in the urine: <11% for hydrocodone after codeine administration and <2.5% for hydromorphone after morphine administration.[53,54,58]

From Smith HS. Opioid metabolism. Mayo Clin Proc. 2009;84(7):613-624; with permission.

(normeperidine), morphine (M6G), and hydromorphone (H3G), may result in accumulation of active metabolites that cause negative adverse effects, such as seizures.[9]

Genetic Considerations

With an increase in access to pharmacogenomics technology, it is possible to evaluate an individual's genetic polymorphisms and potentially to reduce trials of ineffective medications for individual patients. Pharmacogenetics is a relatively new tool in pain medicine but promises a predictive approach to medication therapy choice versus the traditional empirical approach (trial and fail).[14–16]

Gene polymorphism describes the variations in gene structure that lead to variability in ability to metabolize certain medications. Phenotype refers to type of metabolizer, whereas genotype reflects the gene variation.[16,17]

CYP2D6 is an example of highly polymorphic gene, in which 4 major allele combinations have yielded 4 major CYP2D6 phenotypes, as described in[13,15] **Table 4.**

Examples

A poor metabolizer (PM) of CYP2D6 substrates prescribed codeine would be predicted to experience poor analgesia/inefficacy because the prodrug codeine is being weakly converted to the active and effective drug morphine. Alternatively, patients who are ultrametabolizers (UM) may experience significantly more adverse effects as well as greater analgesia.

Table 4 Common metabolic variants		
Types of CYP450 Metabolizers		
Phenotype	Genotype	Effect on Medications
NM/normal metabolizers	2 normal alleles	Normal enzyme activity
IM/intermediate metabolizers	1 normal and 1 reduced allele	Reduced enzyme activity
PM/poor metabolizer	2 mutant alleles with limited/no activity	Low or absent enzyme activity
UM/ultrametabolizer	Multiple normal alleles	Increased enzyme activity

(*Data from* Hay L, Dubovsky SL. Understanding the cytochrome P450 isoenzyme system. NEJM Journal Watch. July 1, 1999. Available at: http://www.jwatch.org/jp199907010000019/1999/07/01/understanding-cytochrome-p450-isoenzyme-system and Dean LC. Codeine therapy and CYP2D6 genotype. In: Pratt VM, McLeod HL, Rubinstein WS, et al, eds. Medical Genetics Summaries [Internet]. Bethesda, MD: National Center for Biotechnology Information; 2012-2016. Available at: http://www.ncbi.nlm.nih.gov/books/NBK100662/.)

Fentanyl is metabolized via the CYP3A4 pathway to inactive metabolites. A PM of fentanyl is at higher risk of potential adverse effects because of higher serum concentrations and delayed elimination of the active parent compound. A UM would be more likely to experience poor analgesia.

The clinical implications of phenotypic variation vary depending on the opioid drug. **Tables 5** and **6** show examples of common substrates, inhibitors, and inducers of CYP 2D6, CYP3A4 and also showcase how they may affect common opioids.[15–17]

CYP3A4 inducers and inhibitors will impact concentrations. The following medications listed in **Table 5** may lead to drug-drug interactions with opioids metabolized by the 3A4 system. For example, carbamazepine is an inducer of CYP3A4, which may lead to lower serum levels and reduced analgesia of oxycodone, methadone, tramadol, and fentanyl.

Special Populations

Elderly
The elderly are at increased risk of changes in hepatic and renal function as well as for polypharmacy and drug-drug interactions. Both pharmacokinetic (CYP3A4 inhibitors and substrates) and pharmacodynamic (additive respiratory depression with opioids and benzodiazepines) effects may be more pronounced in this population.[18]

Decline in renal and hepatic function may result in poor elimination of metabolites and an increased risk of adverse effects. Conversely, hepatic dysfunction may reduce activity of CYP450 isoenzymes and conversion of prodrugs, such as hydrocodone or codeine, into their active metabolites, leading to poor efficacy. For example, reduced hepatic expression of CYP2D6 may lead to reduced efficacy of acetaminophen with codeine products.[16,18]

Patients with cognitive impairment because of injury or dementia may be more susceptible to opioids, leading to delirium, hallucinations, or exacerbation of cognitive problems.[18]

Individuals with cardiovascular, cerebrovascular, or respiratory disease are at increased risk for adverse events related to hypotension, bradycardia, and decreased respiratory drive.[18] Caution is required in patients with these comorbid conditions.

Pregnancy/nursing
Concern and close monitoring is advised regarding fetal opioid dependence in utero and management of withdrawal symptoms of the newborn in the postpartum period

Table 5
Cytochrome P450 3A4 substrates inhibitors, and inducers

Substrates

CCBs
- Amlodipine
- Diltiazem
- Felodipine
- Nicardipine
- Nifedipine
- Verapamil

Statins
- Atorvastatin
- Lovastatin
- Simvastatin

Other cardiovascular agents
- Amiodarone
- Digoxin
- Ivabradine
- Quinidine
- Warfarin

Phosphodiesterase inhibitors
- Sildenafil
- Tadalafil

Benzodiazepines
- Alprazolam
- Clonazepam
- Flunitrazepam
- Midazolam
- Triazolam

SSRIs
- Citalopram
- Fluoxetine

Other psychiatric drugs
- Aripiprazole
- Bromocriptine
- Buspirone
- Carbamazepine
- Donepezil
- Haloperidol
- Mirtazapine
- Nefazodone
- Pimozide
- Reboxetine
- Risperidone
- Valproate
- Venlafaxine
- Ziprasidone

Sleep aids
- Zolpidem
- Zopiclone

Antibiotics
- Azithromycin
- Clarithromycin
- Erythromycin
- Oleandomycin

Azole antifungal agents
- Itraconazole
- Ketoconazole

Antiretroviral agents
- Indinavir
- Lopinavir
- Nelfinavir
- Nevirapine
- Ritonavir
- Saquinavir
- Tipranavir

Chemotherapeutic agents
- Cyclophosphamide
- Docetaxel
- Doxorubicin
- Etoposide
- Gefitinib
- Ifosfamide
- Paclitaxel
- Tamoxifen
- Teniposide
- Vinblastine
- Vindesine

Hormonal therapies
- Estradiol
- Ethinyl estradiol
- Levonorgestrel
- Raloxifene
- Testosterone

Inhibitors

Antibiotics
- Ciprofloxacin
- Clarithromycin
- Erythromycin
- Josamycin
- Norfloxacin
- Oleandomycin
- Roxithromycin
- Telithromycin

Azole antifungal agents
- Clotrimazole
- Fluconazole
- Itraconazole
- Ketoconazole
- Miconazole
- Voriconazole

Antiretroviral agents
- Amprenavir
- Atazanavir
- Delavirdine
- Efavirenz
- Indinavir
- Lopinavir
- Ritonavir
- Nelfinavir
- Nevirapine
- Saquinavir
- Tipranavir

CCBs
- Amlodipine
- Diltiazem
- Felodipine
- Nicardipine
- Nifedipine
- Verapamil

Statin
- Simvastatin

Antiarrhythmic agents
- Amiodarone
- Quinidine

Phosphodiesterase inhibitor
- Tadalafil

Psychiatric drugs
- Bromocriptine
- Clonazepam
- Desipramine
- Fluoxetine
- Fluvoxamine
- Haloperidol
- Nefazodone
- Norclomipramine
- Nortriptyline
- Sertraline

Chemotherapeutic agents
- 4-Ipomeanol
- Imatinib
- Irinotecan
- Tamoxifen

Hormonal therapies
- Ethinyl estradiol
- Levonorgestrel
- Raloxifene

Other drugs
- Cimetidine
- Disulfiram
- Methyl-prednisolone
- Phenelzine

Foods
- Bergamottin (grapefruit juice)
- Star fruit

Inducers

Statins
- Atorvastatin
- Fluvastatin
- Lovastatin
- Simvastatin

Antiretroviral agents
- Efavirenz
- Lopinavir
- Nevirapine

Hypnotic agent
- Pentobarbital

Anticonvulsant agents
- Carbamazepine
- Oxcarbazepine
- Phenobarbital
- Phenytoin
- Primidone
- Valproic acid

Food
- Cafestol
- (caffeine)

Abbreviations: CCB, calcium channel blocker; SSRI, selective serotonin reuptake inhibitor.
From Smith HS. Opioid metabolism. Mayo Clin Proc. 2009;84(7):613-624; with permission.

Table 6
Cytochrome P450 2D6 substrates, inhibitors, and inducers

Substrates	Inhibitors	Inducers
Antiarrhythmic agents	Antiarrhythmic agents	Antibiotic
Encainide	Amiodarone	Rifampin
Flecainide	Quinidine	Glucocorticoid
Lidocaine	Antipsychotic agents	Dexamethasone
Mexiletine	Chlorpromazine	
Propafenone	Reduced haloperidol	
Sparteine	Levomepromazine	
β-Blockers	SNRI	
Alprenolol	Duloxetine	
Carvedilol	SSRIs	
Metoprolol	Citalopram	
Propranolol	Escitalopram	
Timolol	Fluoxetine	
Antipsychotic agents	Paroxetine	
Aripiprazole	Sertraline	
Haloperidol	Tricyclic	
Perphenazine	Clomipramine	
Risperidone	Other antidepressant/	
Thioridazine	antianxiolytic agents	
Zuclopenthixol	Bupropion	
SNRIs	Moclobemide	
Duloxetine	Antihistamine	
Venlafaxine	Chlorpheniramine	
SSRIs	Histamine H_2 receptor	
Fluoxetine	antagonists	
Fluvoxamine	Cimetidine	
Paroxetine	Ranitidine	
Tricyclics	Other drugs	
Amitriptyline	Celecoxib	
Amoxapine	Doxorubicin	
Clomipramine	Ritonavir	
Desipramine	Terbinafine	
Doxepin		
Imipramine		
Nortriptyline		
Other drugs		
Amphetamine		
Chlorpheniramine		
Debrisoquine		
Dextromethorphan		
Histamine H_1 receptor		
antagonists		
Metoclopramide		
Phenformin		
Tamoxifen		

Abbreviation: SNRI, serotonin norepinephrine reuptake inhibitor.
From Smith HS. Opioid metabolism. Mayo Clin Proc. 2009;84(7):613-624; with permission.

(neonatal abstinence syndrome). Caution is recommended for nursing mothers who may be ultrarapid metabolizers and using codeine because morphine levels in breast milk may be significantly elevated and can cause neonatal respiratory depression.[19] The prescriber treating pregnant or nursing mothers must be familiar with the effects of opioid medications in this population.

EFFICACY

The utility of opioids in the management of acute pain has been well demonstrated, and opioids remain a mainstay of treatment of acute pain. In clinical practice. However, it is common for the treatment of acute pain to extend to treatment for longer than intended. There is significant interest in preventing the unintended transition from acute to chronic opioid therapy. Evidence of appropriate duration of opioid prescription in incident pain conditions related to trauma, surgery, and acute disease is a current area of intense interest.

The use of opioids in the treatment of chronic pain remains controversial. In recent history, periods of enthusiastic use have been followed by periods of prohibition as the individual and social costs of misuse accumulated. Such periods occurred in England in the 1800s after the introduction of morphine and after the American Civil War and the introduction of the hypodermic needle.

The systematic evaluation of the efficacy of chronic opioid analgesic therapy (COAT) for chronic pain conditions is less than ideal. Studies are generally methodologically limited and of limited duration.

In 2003, Ballantyne and Mao[20] reviewed the current literature regarding efficacy of COAT and reported that most were reports of surveys or uncontrolled case studies. These studies, most of which reported on periods of only a few weeks, tended to support the effectiveness of opioid therapy in reducing pain. However, the investigators concluded there was no evidence to support 2 important questions: (1) Is opioid therapy beneficial in the long term? and (2) Does dose have an effect on efficacy or safety?

Furlan and colleagues[21] reviewed 41 studies of more than 6000 patients in 2006 and concluded that opioids were superior to placebo, but not superior to naproxen or nortriptyline in chronic pain. Strong opioids were associated with a decrease in pain, but not an improvement in function.

Ballantyne and Shin[22] updated the evidence review in 2008 and concluded that evidence from randomized controlled trials showed evidence for statistically significant improvement in pain in both painful arthritides and neuropathic pain, but cautioned that no randomized controlled trial was longer than 32 weeks and most were much shorter. They also noted that in longer observational studies 58% of patients abandoned COAT because of side effects or lack of effectiveness. They raised concern that analgesic effectiveness may be time limited and that withdrawal of medication after loss of pain relief benefits was difficult because of the development of complex opioid dependency.

Additional analyses have continued to show short-term benefit of opioids compared with placebo.[23] However, the first question above, regarding long-term benefits, remains inadequately studied. Chou and colleagues[24] concluded in 2015 that the evidence is insufficient to determine long-term efficacy for greater than 1 year.

Bialas and colleagues[25] published a metaanalysis in 2019 of open-label studies of greater than 26 weeks and suggested that opioids resulted in lower levels of pain and disability in patients with low back pain, arthritis, and neuropathic pain.[13]

At the time of this writing, the Agency for Health Care Research and Quality posted a public draft of a proposed 2020 publication on opioid treatments for chronic pain, which concludes that the evidence shows a small dose-dependent effect on pain for 1 to 3 months when compared with placebo, but not when compared with nonopioid analgesics.[26]

ADVERSE EFFECTS OF CHRONIC OPIOID THERAPY

The most obvious and emergent adverse event associated with opioids is an "overdose": acute opioid toxicity causing either altered functional ability and a subsequent fall or other trauma or respiratory suppression and risk of death or hypoxic injury. Overdose events have been shown to be positively correlated with opioid dose in multiple studies (**Fig. 1**). At the same time, there is no evidence that higher doses of opioids are associated with improved effectiveness. When a clinician is considering dose escalation for a patient on COAT, these are important considerations (see **Fig. 1**).

The impact of opioid dose on overdose events may be in part mediated by sleep-disordered breathing. Studies have identified a dose-dependent relationship between obstructive and central sleep apnea as well as apnea/hypopnea frequency. Doses of opioids greater than 200 MED and low body mass index are associated with increased risk with ataxic breathing being seen in 92% of individuals treated with more than 200 MED.[27]

Kuo and colleagues[28] recently identified risk factors in a chronically disabled population: those with Medicare insurance who are less than 65 years old. In this group, a combination of diagnoses of chronic pain, a history of substance use disorder, and psychiatric comorbidities increased the risk of overdose by more than 23 times.

Concomitant prescription of opioids with benzodiazepines or sedative hypnotics increases risk of overdose in large population-based studies. For example, in a retrospective study of more than 150,000 patients, the relative risk of death for individuals receiving an opioid prescription was 6.4 when a sedative hypnotic was also prescribed and 12.6 when both a skeletal muscle relaxant and a benzodiazepine were coprescribed with an opioid.[29]

It should also be noted that patients are often unaware of or underestimate the risk of overdose. Wilder and colleagues[30] described awareness of risk among veterans

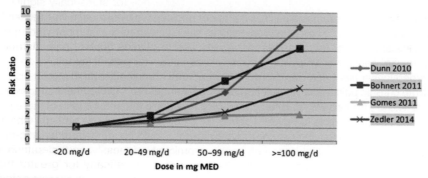

Fig. 1. Risk of overdose event. (*From* Washington State Agency Medical Directors' Group (AMDG). Interagency guideline on prescribing opioids for pain. 3rd ed. Olympia, WA; 2015:12; with permission. Available at http://www.agencymeddirectors.wa.gov/Files/2015AMDGOpioidGuideline.pdf.)

treated with chronic opioids for chronic pain. Of these patients, 70% thought that their risk of overdose was lower than that of the average population. Discussion of risks and benefits of opioids should be informed by the factors described above.

BOWEL DYSFUNCTION

Opioids exert their gastroenterological effects via kappa receptors in the stomach and small bowel and by mu receptors in the small bowel and colon. Constipation is mediated principally via mu receptors. Stimulation of mu receptors causes tonic, nonpropulsive contractions in the small bowel and colon, increased colonic fluid absorption, and dryness of the stool.[31] Constipation is almost universally present to some degree in all patients who use opioids, can reduce quality of life, and is associated with significant health care utilization.

The American Gastroenterological Association published guidelines in 2019 on the management of opioid-induced constipation.[32] They make a strong recommendation for the use of laxatives as a first-line agent for opioid-induced constipation. Laxatives include stool softeners such as docusate sodium, osmotic diuretics such as polyethylene glycol, and stimulants such as senna and bisacodyl. Failure of a combination of at least 2 of these agents is suggested before utilization of peripherally acting mu antagonist agents.

ENDOCRINOPATHIES

The primary mechanism of opioids on the endocrine systems involves suppression of the hypothalamic release of gonadotrophin-releasing hormone and subsequently of luteinizing hormone, follicle-stimulating hormone, and corticotropin, resulting in lower levels of adrenal hormones, such as cortisol and DHEA, and of gonadal hormones, such as testosterone and estradiol.[33]

Although the incidence of opioid-induced endocrinopathy is not clearly known, it is thought to be common. In male patients with symptoms of androgen deficiency, such as depression, fatigue, or reduced libido, or signs such as anemia or osteoporosis, serum testosterone should be checked and repletion considered. Markers of endocrine insufficiency in women are less clear. However, particular attention to bone health is warranted in women treated with opioids.

OPIOID-INDUCED HYPERALGESIA AND COMPLEX OPIOID DEPENDENCY

Opioid-induced hyperalgesia (OIH) is a state of nociceptive hypersensitivity caused by exposure to opioids.[34] This phenomenon has been known to occur in both laboratory and clinical settings. For example, mice exposed to opioids acutely demonstrate a shift toward sensitivity when subsequently presented with painful stimuli.[35]

Hyperalgesia has been demonstrated in patients chronically administered opioids for both chronic pain management and opioid dependence.[36] Clinicians managing patients who are treated with chronic opioids will recognize the phenomena of more pronounced pain responses to incident pain of injury or surgery in those patients who are treated with opioids for chronic pain. Hyperalgesia should be suspected when generalized or ill-defined pain becomes more prominent especially in the setting of increasing opioid dose. Allodynia may also be present.

Several interrelated effects may be present in patients treated with chronic opioids for pain. Tolerance, a decreased analgesic response for a given dose of medication, is known to occur. At the same time, fluctuating blood levels of opioid, a normal occurrence with opioid therapy, may produce periods of subclinical withdrawal. Withdrawal, in addition to producing hyperalgesia, is associated with the phenomenon of hyperkatifeia, an increased sensitivity to emotional distress.[37] At the same time, pronociceptive effects of opioids may emerge. The mechanisms of this phenomenon are poorly understood, but it is thought that at least in part this is mediated through NMDA pathways.

It is likely that many if not most patients treated with opioids chronically experience elements of hyperalgesia and hyperkatifeia in addition to periods of pain reduction and anxiety reduction related to opioids. In recognition of this, the term "complex opioid dependency" has been introduced.[38]

Patients treated with opioids for a long period of time may exhibit complex opioid dependency. Complex opioid dependency is not equivalent to an opioid use disorder and involves neurologic changes that can have complex and profound influences on function and quality of life. Changes in pain state and emotional state may become tied more to current opioid blood level than to the factors that would otherwise normally influence pain and mood. Whether these neurologic changes are reversible is not fully known.

The optimal management for complex opioid dependency is also not clearly known. The goals of treatment include restoration of internal homeostasis, management of the underlying pain for which the opioid was initially prescribed, and mitigation of the adverse effects of the opioid. When hyperalgesia or other adverse effects of opioid therapy predominate, reduction or elimination of the opioid may be helpful. However, this is a difficult process, and in usual practice, patients tapered from opioids with persistent or worsened pain may not tolerate the process and may not be offered alternatives to tapering. There is some reason to think that a transition to long-acting opioids with NMDA antagonist activity, such as methadone, may offer improved efficacy when OIH is present.[39] There is also evidence that buprenorphine may be effective in treating patients with opioid-induced hypersensitivity.[40]

Emerging guidelines suggest a practical approach to management of complex opioid dependency in the setting of persistent pain. As an important example, the US Department of Health and Human Services provided recommendations in October 2019.[41] When benefits outweigh risks of the therapy, continued therapy and monitoring are recommended. When the contrary is true, tapering, generally slow tapering, is recommended. For those patients who do not tolerate tapering because of distress or increased pain, medication-assisted treatment with buprenorphine, potentially indefinitely, is recommended. The hope is that this approach is both safer and potentially more stable in regard to analgesia than continued management with pure agonist medications. Further studies as to the effectiveness of this approach in the population of patients with persistent pain and chronic opioid analgesic exposure are important.

SUMMARY

Opioids are a primary endogenous mediator of pain and reward. They have been used since prehistoric times and remain one of the most commonly used medicines today. Although the use of opioids in chronic therapy may be associated with reduced reports of pain severity; however, benefits in terms of improved function and quality of life are not uniformly present. People treated with opioids for a prolonged period may develop a state of complex opioid dependency, which further complicates management of persistent pain. Improving outcomes for these individuals is a focus of intense current interest.

DISCLOSURE

The authors have nothing to disclose.

REFERENCES

1. Brownstein MJ. A brief history of opiates, opioid peptides, and opioid receptors. Proc Natl Acad Sci U S A 1993;90(12):5391.
2. Kalant H. Opium revisited: a brief review of its nature, composition, non-medical use and relative risks 1. Addiction 1997;92(3):267–77.
3. Brook K, Bennett J, Desai SP. The chemical history of morphine: an 8000-year journey, from resin to de-novo synthesis. J Anesth Hist 2017;3(2):50–5.
4. Moradi M, Esmaeili S, Shoar S, et al. Use of oxycodone in pain management. Anesthesiol Pain Med 2012;1(4):262.
5. Squire LR, Dronkers N, Baldo J. Encyclopedia of neuroscience. Elsevier; 2009.
6. Chavkin C. The therapeutic potential of kappa-opioids for treatment of pain and addiction. Neuropsychopharmacology 2011;36(1):369–70.
7. Pradhan AA, Befort K, Nozaki C, et al. The delta opioid receptor: an evolving target for the treatment of brain disorders. Trends Pharmacol Sci 2011;32(10): 581–90.
8. Leppert W, Krajnik M, Wordliczek J. Delivery systems of opioid analgesics for pain relief: a review. Curr Pharm Des 2013;19(41):7271–93.
9. Schumacher M, Basbaum A, Naidu R. Opioid analgesics and antagonists. Basic and clinical pharmacology. 11th edition. McGraw-Hill; 2009.
10. Garland EL, Froeliger B, Zeidan F, et al. The downward spiral of chronic pain, prescription opioid misuse, and addiction: cognitive, affective, and neuropsychopharmacologic pathways. Neurosci Biobehav Rev 2013;37(10):2597–607.
11. Trescot AM, Datta S, Lee M, et al. Opioid pharmacology. Pain Physician 2008; 11(2 Suppl):S133–53.
12. Smith HS. Opioid metabolism. Mayo Clin Proc 2009;84(7):613–24. Elsevier.
13. Holmquist GL. Opioid metabolism and effects of cytochrome P450. Pain Med 2009;10(suppl_1):S20–9.
14. Richmeier S, Lee J. Genetic testing in pain medicine–the future is coming. Practical pain management 2017. Available at: http://www.practicalpainmanagement. com/treatments/genetic-testing-pain-medicine-future-coming.
15. Overholser BR, Foster DR. Opioid pharmacokinetic drug-drug interactions. Am J Manag Care 2011;17:S276–87.
16. Schuft K. Pharmacogenomics: effect of gene variability on pain management. Wolters Kluwer; 2018. Available at: https://www.wolterskluwercdi.com/blog/ pharmacogenomics-effect-gene-variability-pain-management/.
17. Agarwal D, Udoji MA, Trescot A. Genetic testing for opioid pain management: a primer. Pain Ther 2017;6(1):93–105.
18. Lynch T. Management of drug-drug interactions: considerations for special populations–focus on opioid use in the elderly and long term care. Am J Manag Care 2011;17:S293–8.
19. King S, Forbes K, Hanks G, et al. A systematic review of the use of opioid medication for those with moderate to severe cancer pain and renal impairment: a European Palliative Care Research Collaborative opioid guidelines project. Palliat Med 2011;25(5):525–52.
20. Ballantyne JC, Mao J. Opioid therapy for chronic pain. N Engl J Med 2003; 349(20):1943–53.

21. Furlan AD, Sandoval JA, Mailis-Gagnon A, et al. Opioids for chronic noncancer pain: a meta-analysis of effectiveness and side effects. CMAJ 2006;174(11): 1589–94.
22. Ballantyne JC, Shin NS. Efficacy of opioids for chronic pain: a review of the evidence. Clin J pain 2008;24(6):469–78.
23. Meske DS, Lawal OD, Elder H, et al. Efficacy of opioids versus placebo in chronic pain: a systematic review and meta-analysis of enriched enrollment randomized withdrawal trials. J Pain Res 2018;11:923.
24. Chou R, Turner JA, Devine EB, et al. The effectiveness and risks of long-term opioid therapy for chronic pain: a systematic review for a National Institutes of Health Pathways to Prevention Workshop. Ann Intern Med 2015;162(4):276–86.
25. Bialas P, Maier C, Klose P, et al. Efficacy and harms of long-term opioid therapy in chronic non-cancer pain: systematic review and meta-analysis of open-label extension trials with a study duration ≥26 weeks. Eur J Pain 2019;24(2):265–78.
26. Agency for Healthcare Research and Quality [
27. Cheatle MD, Webster LR. Opioid therapy and sleep disorders: risks and mitigation strategies. Pain Med 2015;16(suppl_1):S22–6.
28. Kuo Y-F, Raji MA, Goodwin JS. Association of disability with mortality from opioid overdose among US Medicare adults. JAMA Netw open 2019;2(11):e1915638.
29. Garg RK, Fulton-Kehoe D, Franklin GM. Patterns of opioid use and risk of opioid overdose death among Medicaid patients. Med Care 2017;55(7):661–8.
30. Wilder CM, Miller SC, Tiffany E, et al. Risk factors for opioid overdose and awareness of overdose risk among veterans prescribed chronic opioids for addiction or pain. J Addict Dis 2016;35(1):42–51.
31. Dorn S, Lembo A, Cremonini F. Opioid-induced bowel dysfunction: epidemiology, pathophysiology, diagnosis, and initial therapeutic approach. Am J Gastroenterol Suppl 2014;2(1):31.
32. Crockett SD, Greer KB, Heidelbaugh JJ, et al. American Gastroenterological Association Institute guideline on the medical management of opioid-induced constipation. Gastroenterology 2019;156(1):218–26.
33. Colameco S, Coren JS. Opioid-induced endocrinopathy. J Am Osteopath Assoc 2009;109(1):20–5.
34. Marion Lee M, Sanford Silverman M, Hans Hansen M, et al. A comprehensive review of opioid-induced hyperalgesia. Pain Physician 2011;14:145–61.
35. Mao J. Opioid-induced abnormal pain sensitivity: implications in clinical opioid therapy. Pain 2002;100(3):213–7.
36. Hay JL, White JM, Bochner F, et al. Hyperalgesia in opioid-managed chronic pain and opioid-dependent patients. J Pain 2009;10(3):316–22.
37. Grandy J. A clinical correlation made between opioid-induced hyperalgesia and hyperkatifeia with brain alterations induced by long-term prescription opioid use. J Neurosci 2012;2(2):1–11.
38. Ballantyne JC, Sullivan MD, Kolodny A. Opioid dependence vs addiction: a distinction without a difference? Arch Intern Med 2012;172(17):1342–3.
39. Axelrod DJ, Reville B. Using methadone to treat opioid-induced hyperalgesia and refractory pain. J Opioid Manag 2007;3(2):113–4.
40. Koppert W, Ihmsen H, Körber N, et al. Different profiles of buprenorphine-induced analgesia and antihyperalgesia in a human pain model. Pain 2005; 118(1–2):15–22.
41. HHS guide for clinicians on the appropriate dosage reduction or discontinuation of long-term opioid analgesics. In: Services USDoHaH, editor. 2019.

Moving?

Make sure your subscription moves with you!

To notify us of your new address, find your **Clinics Account Number** (located on your mailing label above your name), and contact customer service at:

Email: journalscustomerservice-usa@elsevier.com

800-654-2452 (subscribers in the U.S. & Canada)
314-447-8871 (subscribers outside of the U.S. & Canada)

Fax number: 314-447-8029

Elsevier Health Sciences Division
Subscription Customer Service
3251 Riverport Lane
Maryland Heights, MO 63043

*To ensure uninterrupted delivery of your subscription, please notify us at least 4 weeks in advance of move.

Printed and bound by CPI Group (UK) Ltd, Croydon, CR0 4YY

03/10/2024

01040408-0010